the Potato Reset

WEIGHT LOSS & RECIPE GUIDE BY JEANNINE ELDER

ISBN # 978-1986840767

Potato Reset Praise

High Carb Hannah
Author of *Lean & Clean*

"The Potato Reset is a great guide for anyone looking to lose weight, regain their health or press the reset button on their palate. I know from experience how amazing a potato diet can be for you. Being able to eat until your full everyday and having energy to tackle life all while losing weight is the definition of a great diet to me. This book will give you all the tools to get back on track and some amazing recipes so that you never feel deprived."

Chef A.J.
Author of *Unprocessed* and
The Secrets to Ultimate Weight Loss

"A recipe book of all potato recipes is long overdue. Potatoes are not only the most satiating food on the planet, but by far, one of the most nutritious. Whether you are a full blown food addict, someone who needs to lose a few pounds or just someone who would like to eat healthier, The Potato Reset is just what the doctored ordered."

Andrew Spudfit Taylor
Author of *DIY Spudfit*

"The Potato Reset is beautiful in its simplicity, beautiful in its design and beautiful in its message. The information and inspiration in this book will give you everything you need to get started down a new, healthful path in both body and mind."

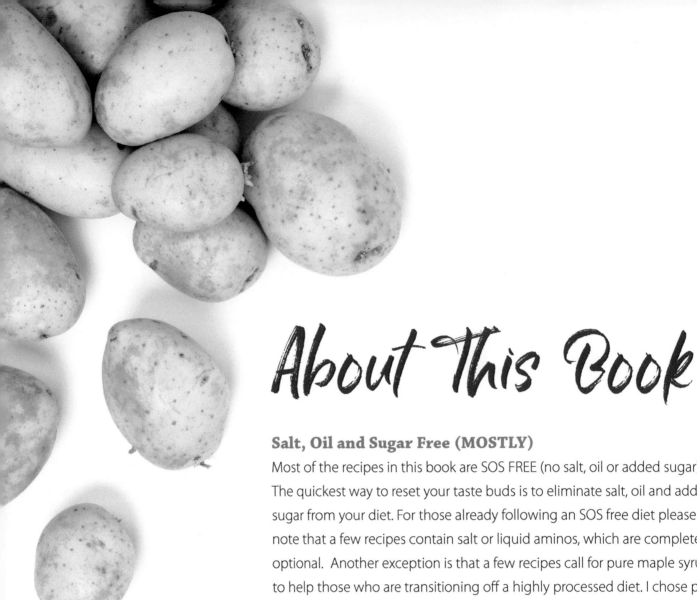

About This Book

Salt, Oil and Sugar Free (MOSTLY)

Most of the recipes in this book are SOS FREE (no salt, oil or added sugar). The quickest way to reset your taste buds is to eliminate salt, oil and added sugar from your diet. For those already following an SOS free diet please note that a few recipes contain salt or liquid aminos, which are completely optional. Another exception is that a few recipes call for pure maple syrup to help those who are transitioning off a highly processed diet. I chose pure maple syrup because it's easy to find just about anywhere – feel free to omit, replace with date syrup or homemade date paste.

Serving Sizes

Serving sizes are a rough estimate. The point of The Potato Reset is to learn to trust your hunger signals, therefore I give rough estimates on the serving sizes. I don't know what portion sizes everyone will need or if they are sharing the meal with someone. After a week on this plan you will get a better idea for how much you need to eat to feel satisfied.

Bonus Printables

There are some helpful reference pages in this book that you may want to put on your fridge. Instead of ripping them out of this book go to **potatoreset.com/bonus** to download and print.

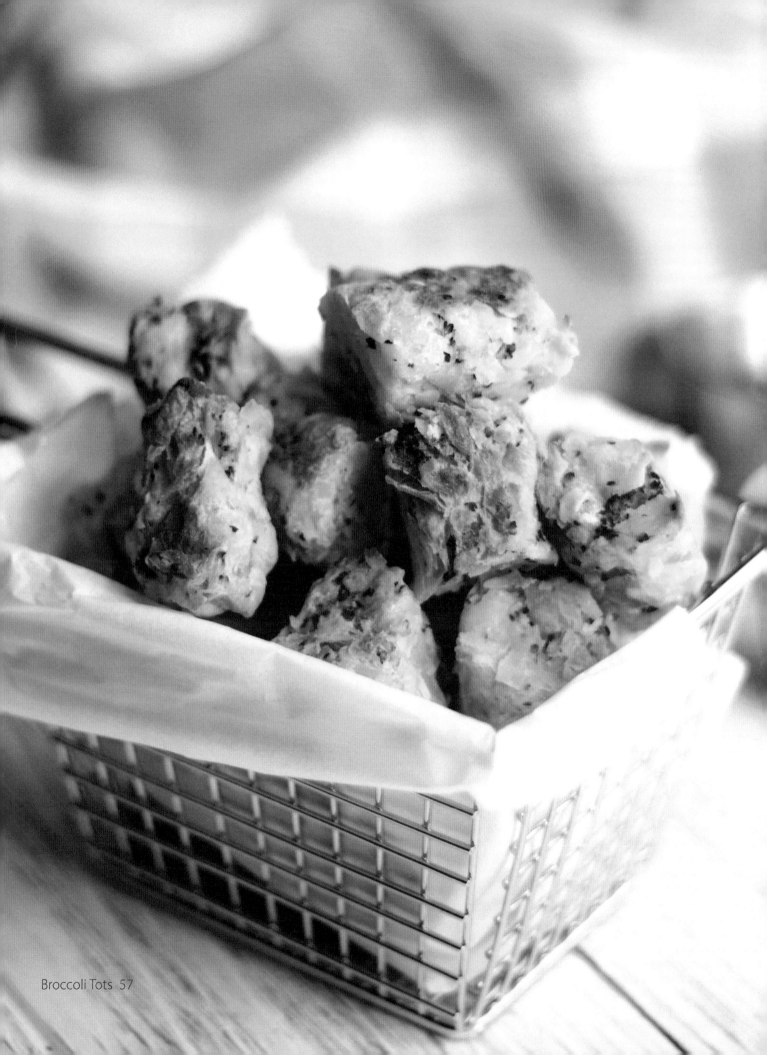

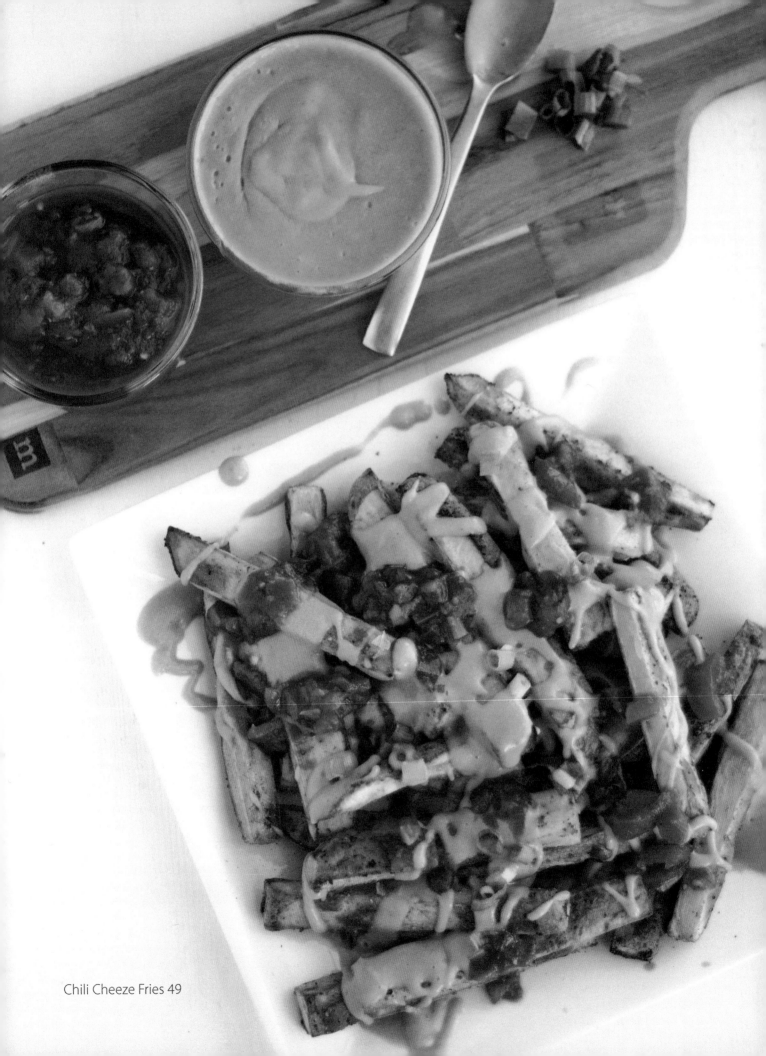

Chili Cheeze Fries 49

Table of Contents

Information

Meal Planning

Sauce & Spice Guide

Batch Cooking Recipes

Slimming Soups

Finger Food

Dat Crunch

Comfort Food

Dessert

How I Got Here

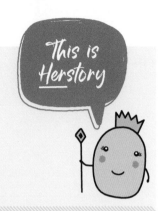

This is Herstory

MY NAME IS JEANNINE, affectionately known as Potato Wisdom on YouTube. In the past eight months I've completely changed my relationship with food and lost over 33 pounds – without driving myself crazy or feeling deprived. I feel vibrant and happy, despite having gallstones and Hashimoto's Thyroiditis. This is a stark comparison to where I was ten years ago.

In my early 30s I was almost 100 pounds heavier, sleeping over 15 hours a day and suffering from debilitating depression, memory loss and brain fog. This is my story about how I went from a zombie to a happy, healthy woman in her 40s.

After many years of being brushed off, or told it was "just depression" by medical doctors, as well as being accused by my (now ex) husband that I was "faking it" so I could take time off work — I finally received an explanation for my symptoms. I was diagnosed with Hashimoto's Thyroiditis, an autoimmune condition that causes the immune system to attack the thyroid, leaving behind an under active thyroid gland, full of nodules. The result is hypothyroidism, and the only treatment, according to doctors, is thyroid replacement therapy.

My diagnosis came from an endocrinologist, a doctor that specializes in glandular diseases. During my first endocrinologist appointment, she had me step on the scale: I saw 260 pounds staring back at me. How is that possible? I was 240 pounds just a month ago when I weighed in for my annual physical. I hadn't changed my diet or activity levels. I didn't realize it was even possible to put on that kind of weight without stuffing my face with entire bags of cookies or doubling up on drive-thru meals. According to the BMI chart, at five feet four inches

tall and 260 pounds I was morbidly obese. Not just obese but morbidly obese. Those words echoed through my brain fog and punched my heart.

This is not precisely where my weight or health problems started. I always had health ailments as a child: ear infections, eczema, colds, flus and mono. And I can't really pinpoint when my weight was actually a real physical problem. The earliest memory of being "fat" was when I was 8 years old,

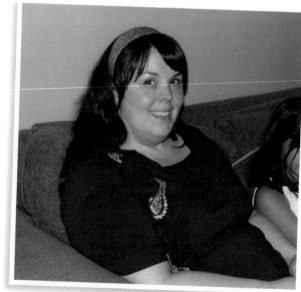

Me at the age of 33 and 1.5 years after my thyroid treatment started. I was approximately 230 lbs here.

sitting with my friend in lawn chairs in my front yard after playing in the sprinkler. We looked down at our slightly rounded kid-bellies and counted our rolls, while purposely hunched over in order to make said belly rolls. It was a gradual process of fat-observations like this and kids making fun of me for having an ounce more padding than them that led to eventually believing I was fat and ugly.

As an adult looking through photos of my childhood and teenage years, I can't find any evidence of a fat girl. If I could time travel, I'd go back and slap my younger self silly — scratch that — I'd hug her, and tell her she's beautiful. And I would tell her to eat healthier, not that she would have listened. While I wasn't an obese child, this is where my lifelong love of junk and processed food began. Other than fruit, everything I ate was processed and I hated vegetables.

Besides dieting a few times in my late teens to lose some vanity pounds here and there, my weight struggles really started in my 20s after graduating college and working a full time desk job. It's simple math really: junk food + desk job + suburbitis (needing a car to get everywhere) = weight gain. My weight fluctuated within 20 pounds depending on my gym attendance and eating habits. My highest weight hovered around 170 pounds. Or so I thought.

I was 24 when I moved to Vancouver and the reality of how out of shape I was smacked me in the face, hard. Going from suburbia to city life was like suddenly marathoning everyday. I went from driving everywhere to walking just about everywhere. Even when I took the bus I still had to walk to get there.

Death became a regular fantasy, the idea of no longer living seemed like the only way out of this.

After joining a gym I was surprised when my body assessment revealed that I was 194 pounds and 41% fat. Another new reality: almost half of my body was made up of fat and I was almost 200 pounds.

After nine months of "eating right" and hitting the gym six days a week I just barely squeezed off half a pound a week on average – around 25 pounds total. I fluctuated between 185 and 165 for the next five or so years. I found the Atkins diet when I was looking for ways to lose enough weight to look presentable in my belly dance costume, within a couple of months I lost 15 pounds and got to my lowest adult weight of 150 pounds. Of course, it wasn't sustainable and I gained it all back, and more, when I resumed my normal way of eating.

Within a few months of my Atkins craze I started to notice an increased sensitivity to alcohol which caused major fluid retention and face puffiness (from one drink!) The mild depression and low energy that was dismissed by my doctor a few years ago had worsened. That's the time when my doctor, informed me that I had "sub clinical" hypothyroidism and that it was "nothing to worry about".

"Nothing to worry about" turned out to become suicidal depression and an inability to perform at my job. After being told I was "just depressed" I became increasingly unstable because I thought depression was a self-induced problem that I just needed to get over. Death became a regular fantasy, the idea of no longer living seemed like the only way out of this. To add another blow to my self-esteem, I was let go from my job after applying for medical leave. Despite reassurance that it was a corporate restructuring issue and that there was zero issue with my job performance – no one could convince me otherwise, not even the generous severance payout. I didn't know it then but it's exactly what I needed.

It was a couple of months after becoming unemployed that I was diagnosed with Hashimoto's at the age of 32. If it wasn't for finding a competent doctor I'm not sure I would be alive today. My endocrinologist put me on thyroid medication straight away then sent me off for a thyroid ultrasound and a biopsy to screen for cancer. The biopsy results where inconclusive, so they couldn't rule out cancer without surgically removing the suspicious nodule. I was given a thyroid cancer pamphlet and reassured that thyroid is the best kind of cancer to get because it grows so slowly (oh yay!). From then on my nodules would be monitored for growth through ultrasounds.

Every six weeks my blood was tested and medication increased until my thyroid levels (TSH) satisfied my endocrinologist. A year later she sat across from me at her desk, beaming with pride, my TSH was 2.0 – "this is perfect!".

I wasn't feeling *perfect* but I felt better than death, which was a huge improvement. And I wasn't quite ready to go back to work but I didn't actually have a choice, I needed the money. After a year and a half of not working I was suddenly faced with the reality of having to actually dress this 260 pound body in something other than lounging-around-the-house clothes and do something other than lounging around the house.

As I walked into the plus-sized store I felt humiliated and I doubted that I would be able to find outfits not resembling something my grandmother would wear to a nice night out at the Chinese Buffet or the professional banker lady pant-suit with an oversized jacket to keep it all

hidden. I imagined myself wearing my hair big and starting a collection of shiny metal brooches. To my surprise, I walked out of that store smiling ear-to-ear with three very stylish outfits! I was never so happy to be wrong.

Soon after starting my new job the weight began to come off without effort. I lost around 40 pounds in six months despite the fact that I was still eating the same way I normally ate (processed with a pinch of healthy.) After that I had to put some effort into it.

It was around this time that I started dating someone who treated me like a queen, and I was on cloud nine. If I had any Hashimoto's symptoms at this point, I probably wouldn't have noticed. I was falling in love with the most amazing man on the planet and had the energy of a nine-year-old on Christmas morning.

I was motivated to continue with losing weight and I wanted to get serious about it, so I hired a

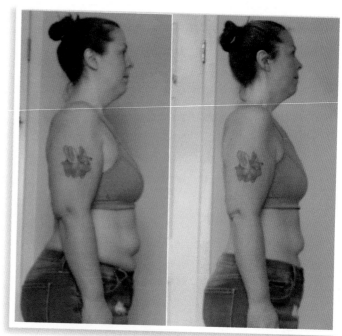

On the left I was in February 2017 on the right August 2017, all while eating plenty of potatoes.

personal trainer. He had me eating 1,300 calories a day while putting me through intense training sessions and I lost over 30 pounds in three months. I do not recommend this method because extreme caloric restriction and intense exercise are both very stressful on the body. I believe this stress is what caused my Hashimoto's symptoms to make another appearance in my life.

Miraculously I kept some of that 30 pounds off and maintained for about a year. Then I married my best friend and gained a little more – it's true that we eat more with good company. About a year into our marriage my weight crept back up to 200 pounds. Soon after we switched to a plant-based diet after watching the documentary "Forks Over Knives".

I lost 25 pounds in the first 6 months of eating plant based. But I gained that 25 pounds back after discovering processed vegan products and vegan junk food. When the scale tipped 200 again I decided to put an end to my ever expanding body – I got back down to 171 between January and August 2014 by restricting calories (a.k.a. whining to my husband every night that "I'm still hungry".)

That summer, I found this slim and vibrant woman on YouTube who goes by the name of Freelee the Banana Girl. I binged-watched her videos, fascinated by her ability to eat endless amounts of fruit, rice and potatoes. I started following her Raw Till Four way of eating: fruit for breakfast and lunch, then a cooked carb-rich low fat meal for dinner. That's when I started a YouTube channel to document my health journey. I felt great on this lifestyle and I looked leaner but I never really felt satisfied from large fruit meals or gigantic smoothies.

Raw Till Four didn't keep me away from junk food completely, but it was the healthiest I've ever eaten in my life, and my thyroid was functioning so well that my doctor decreased my medication. Unfortunately she reduced too much too soon, I felt symptomatic and was put back on my regular dose. Five months later she had me try again and was successful, I've been on the lowered dose ever since. Both times when the medication was reduced I gained five pounds that never came off. I gained more weight after this but it was no fault of my thyroid.

> I knew that I needed to stay away from junk food in order to achieve long term and sustainable weight loss and health.

I knew that I needed to stay away from junk food in order to achieve long term sustainable weight loss and health. In October 2016, after spending a weekend in Portland with three inspiring women (Heather, Chef AJ and her bestie Shayda) with an unwavering commitment to healthy eating, I was finally ready to face the reality that I had a junk food addiction, and that I was stuck in the pleasure trap – I used food for pleasure rather than nourishment.

Back at home, I weighed myself for the first time in months. I was almost 210 pounds! I was ready for change. I made it through the holiday season without eating junk, thanks to High Carb Hannah's Lean & Clean meal plan. I managed to lose 7 or so pounds during the most tempting junk-filled time of year!

I had been wanting to do a potato-diet challenge for a couple of years but was afraid to try it – the fear of failure held me back. The previous year I watched High Carb Hannah do a 30-Day Potato Cleanse where she ate only potatoes and veggies

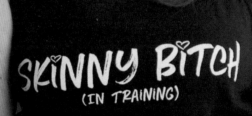

and that same year, "Spud Fit" Andrew Taylor ate only potatoes for the whole year. In February 2017, I decided to take on the challenge and do an all-potato diet for the entire month and shared the experience on YouTube.

The reason I chose to start with potatoes-only was because I didn't like vegetables unless they were hidden in a recipe and drowned in sauce. Adding vegetables would have led to quitting real fast.

I hoped that eating potatoes for a month would reset my taste buds enough to tolerate more veggies. And it worked! For the first time in my life, at the age of 41, I was able to eat broccoli without gagging. For the 2nd and 3rd months I added vegetables along with my potatoes.

By the fourth month I was slowly incorporating more whole plant foods such as fruit, rice and quinoa. Then later small quantities of nuts and seeds and lastly, lentils and beans – I did this in order of what was best for my digestion. In eight months I have lost over 33 pounds, eating a lot of potatoes. This is the first time in a very long time that I've been in the 160s. What amazes me is that I lost 33 pounds without counting calories or feeling deprived. And most importantly, I reset my taste buds and improved my relationship with food. I went from hating most vegetables to tolerating vegetables! Do I slip up and eat processed food? Sometimes, but I rarely overdo it and it's not as enjoyable as it used to be.

What amazes me is that I lost 33 pounds without counting calories or feeling deprived.

You will be amazed how much better real food tastes after following the guidelines in this book. I have another 30 or so pounds to go and plan to get there with the power of the potato. I'm so excited to have you join me on this journey!

Connect with Me

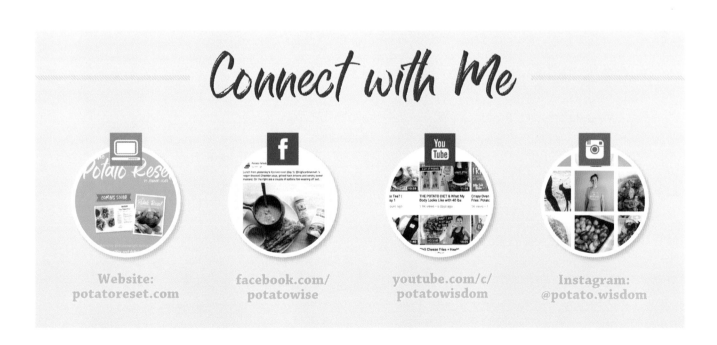

Website:
potatoreset.com

facebook.com/
potatowise

youtube.com/c/
potatowisdom

Instagram:
@potato.wisdom

Get Ready to Reset!

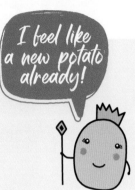

I feel like a new potato already!

READY TO GET STARTED? It's just like planning a party, a potato party! I want you to get excited about this and most importantly I want you to be prepared. Decide on a start date and time frame that is doable for you, set goals, tell everyone and maybe even find a potato ~~buddy~~ spuddy. Let's get our potato sacks on and hop down the path to resetting!

Set Goals

Seeing the scale going down is exciting, but there is so much more to the Potato Reset than weight loss. We can get so wrapped up with the numbers that mini-victories don't get the attention they deserve.

These mini-victories can be pivotal in keeping us motivated when the number on the scale isn't moving. I encourage you to write a list of non-scale goals you would like to achieve while on the Potato Reset and check in with your list each week.

Examples:
- This tummy bloat has got to go
- Get rid of junk food cravings
- Stop nighttime snacking
- Reduce medication
- Clear up acne
- Be able to say "no" to Mom's baking
- Improve my relationship with food
- I want my clothes to fit better
- Reduce joint pain
- Sleep better
- Learn to love vegetables
- Have more energy
- Be naturally drawn to healthy food
- Improve my cholesterol
- Improve blood pressure

Take Measurements & Photos

A day or two before your start date, take some full-body, "before" photos (front, side, and back) with as much skin as you're comfortable showing – perhaps wearing a sports bra and shorts or a tank top and cropped tights.

Next, take your measurements and write them down. Here's what I've been measuring: neck, bust, below bust, waist (smallest part), belly button area, hips, thighs, knees, calves and ankles. Measure as much or as little as you like. And if the scale is not a problem for you, weigh yourself first thing in the morning on your first day.

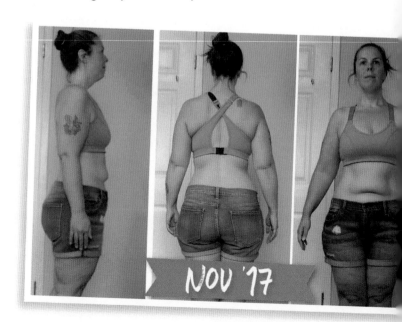

NOV '17

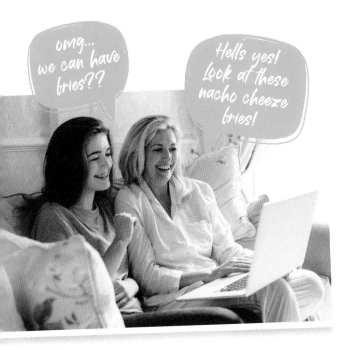

Tell Everyone

Mark your start date on the calendar and begin to mentally prepare yourself. Tell everyone you live with that you're doing a little potato experiment and what it's all about. This will help them understand what you might need from them to get through this. For me, telling everyone who was willing to listen made me want to follow through and complete my challenge. Share your daily meals on InstaGram or YouTube if you're up for it – be sure to use the hashtag #potatoreset so we can all find each other.

Find a Spuddy

Your best-case scenario is to find a local buddy, such as a friend, coworker, or family member to do this with you. If that's not possible, I recommend you share your experience online and perhaps even find an accountability partner through social media. I personally met a lot of "spuddies" through Instagram just by sharing my potato photos. There are over 14,000 potential spuddies in my Facebook group: **facebook.com/groups/thepotatodiet**

Get Inspired

Find a potato diet veteran who inspires you by searching the keyword #spudfit #potatodiet #potatoreset #potatocleanse on Instagram. Or do a YouTube search for "potato diet" "potato reset" or "potato cleanse". Some of my favorites on YouTube are Spud Fit Andrew Taylor, Debt Free Dayna, High Carb Hannah, Jordon Shrinks and Potato Wisdom (I can toot my own horn, right?).

Buy a 10-lb Bag of Potatoes

During the week before your official start date get yourself a 10-lb bag of potatoes and divide it into 10 equal parts. Now you know what a pound of potatoes looks like. Eat a potato meal everyday, try out the recipes, and see how many meals a 10-lb bag lasts you. This should give you an estimate of how many pounds you eat per meal and how many potatoes you should buy for the first week. During my potato diet, I ate around four pounds of potatoes per day (28 lbs of potatoes per week.)

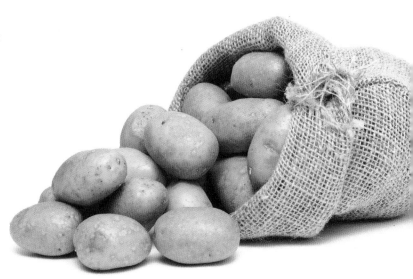

What is the Potato Reset?

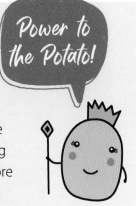

Power to the Potato!

THE POTATO RESET is essentially the Potato Cleanse, re-branded, to better describe what this plan is about. The Potato Cleanse made it's debut in January 2016 when High Carb Hannah decided she wanted to do a mono diet – sometimes known as an "island" diet, where you eat only one kind of food for set amount of days. The most popular mono diet is "Banana Island". Hannah chose potatoes because she knew they are one of the most nutrient dense and satisfying foods on the planet which makes them ideal for weight loss. To make the plan more interesting and nutrient dense she added in non-starchy vegetables.

More of a Reset than a Cleanse

I chose to name this book The Potato Reset because it's not a cleanse in the traditional sense — we aren't juicing, water fasting or taking herbs to clean out our digestive tract, and it's not a quick fix, like many cleanses are intended to be. The term "cleanse" brings back memories of herbal cleanses I've done in the past, the kind that evoked sudden exorcisms of all the evil that lay dormant in my colon. While this plan may have a gentle cleansing effect on your colon, it's not likely to lead to sudden trips to the bathroom.

The Potato Reset helps to reset your taste buds, reset your relationship with food, and reset your ability to trust your hunger signals. This plan is for anyone who wants to lose weight in a healthy way without calorie counting or feeling restricted and hungry all the time. It's also for those who want to stop obsessive calorie counting, those who want to learn to trust their body again and those who want to get a handle on their junk food addiction.

The Basics

While on the Potato Reset plan we only consume potatoes, sweet potatoes, non-starchy vegetables, spices and plant-based sauces. We avoid overt fats such as oil, butter, cheese, sour cream, mayo, nuts, seeds, avocado and even tofu. We avoid beans, lentils and other legumes. See page 19 for a full list of foods allowed on the Potato Reset.

The following are some of the questions I hear on a regular basis from people who want to know more about the specific process that went into designing this plan.

Why Potatoes?

Potatoes are satisfying, versatile, full of minerals and vitamins, rich in fiber and even provide more than enough protein. They are the perfect food for weight loss and who doesn't love potatoes?

"One 5-ounce baked potato has 150 calories. An active man may burn 3000 calories a day and a woman 2300 calories a day. That means the man would have to eat 20 potatoes and the woman 15 potatoes or they would lose weight. That's 5 to 7 large potatoes per meal, three times a day – a big

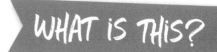

dent in even the hardiest appetite – especially considering potatoes are among the most satisfying of all foods." – drmcdougall.com

Why Low Fat?

The plan purposely excludes overt fats, meaning no added fats. That means no oil, butter, cheese, sour cream, nuts, seeds, avocado and tofu. There is a small amount of naturally occurring fat in all vegetables, and unless you have very little fat left on your body you need not worry about missing out on essential fatty acids. The reason for this is because fats are calorically dense and not as filling as non-starchy vegetables and potatoes. Eating low-calorie dense foods allows us to fill up and feel satisfied without having to worry about over consuming calories. This means you can trust your body to eat the right amount of food without having to weigh, measure and count calories!

Why Minimize Salt & Sugar?

There is a reason why restaurant food is extremely high in sodium, because it tastes great and keeps us coming back for more. We want to understimulate the taste buds so that we eat to natural satiation. We achieve this by keeping salt and sugar to a minimum. This allows your tastes to reset and actually taste the actual food. I was amazed when I began to enjoy oven baked fries without any sauce, salt or seasonings. And even more amazed when some of my favorite junk foods no longer tasted as good as I remember, some even caused me to feel nauseated after a few bites.

Am I Hungry or Craving?

The magical potato is responsible for teaching me the difference between real hunger and cravings. I realized that for most of my life, what I thought was hunger really wasn't hunger: it was either boredom, hormones, stress, or lack-of-sleep hunger. In other words I was eating to satisfy cravings, not to satisfy actual hunger. A very simple way to test if you're experiencing hunger or cravings: does a plain potato or vegetable sound good to you in that moment? If the answer is no, you're not hungry. Several times during my first week on the potato diet I thought I felt hungry, but wanted something other than a damn potato — "I don't want a potato I want something else!"— but soon, fruit never looked more appealing and beautiful in my life.

What About Beans, Rice and Quinoa?

Why are these healthy foods not included on the plan? While all these foods are healthy, the simple reason they are not included is because this is the potato diet and not the bean/rice/quinoa diet. Just because a food is excluded from this plan does not mean it's "bad", it just didn't make the cut. I encourage you to incorporate these foods into your diet after the Potato Reset.

If potatoes cause stomach upset for you, peeling your potatoes and experiment with different varieties. It may mean all you eat is sweet potatoes and golden potatoes.

Does This Plan Require a Lot of Exercise?

Absolutely not. If you are currently sedentary I suggest adding in some light exercise such as walking and/or yoga. For the first couple of months I was only walking around 20 minutes per day, occasionally 40 minutes. If you're already active, continue with your regular exercise routine if it's not rigorous (such as training for a marathon).

Potato Reset Guidelines

POTATOES ARE THE STAR OF THE SHOW and your main source of calories. Some of the most common varieties include russet, white, yellow and red. And of course we can't forget the sweet potato and many varieties available from yellow to orange (typically called yams) to purple. No other starchy foods are allowed – no corn, beans, rice, or grains. You can have as many non-starchy vegetables as you like (see list below). You can eat the potatoes any way you like – mashed, baked, hash browns, potato pancakes, fries, soups, stews, etc. Be creative!. You can also eat potatoes only, if you wish.

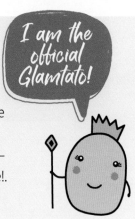

I am the official Glamtato!

Condiments

Homemade sauces are the best, because you can control how much sodium and sweetness goes into it. But don't stress if you can't make your own, just don't drench your taters in store-bought sauces, as they tend to be high in sodium and processed sugar.

Avoid heavily processed sugars and artificial sweeteners. One exception to the rule, to keep you sane while you wean off sweet cravings, you can use 100% pure maple syrup or date syrup/puree – two tablespoons max per day – preferably as part of a sauce recipe and not straight-up. For sauce shopping tips and recipes see pages 30 - 35.

Spices

Use as much salt-free and sugar-free spices and herbs as you'd like. And because every vegan will ask: yes, you can use nutritional yeast flakes.

Use salt sparingly, sprinkle on your food after cooking – do not cook with salt. For spice shopping tips, homemade herbal salt and spice blend recipes see pages 28 - 29.

Drinks & Liquids

For hydration your best bet is water, you may also have unsweetened sparkling water and herbal tea. If you can't stand to drink plain water add fresh lemon juice, lime juice or sliced cucumbers to your water. Coffee and caffeine teas are permitted but please avoid using sweeteners and dairy – I recommend a small amount of unsweetened non-dairy milk such as unsweetened almond milk in place of milk/creamer.

For potato mashing and soups I recommend having on hand unsweetened non-dairy milk and low sodium or no-salt-added vegetable broth.

Unlimited Non-Starchy Veggies

If you love veggies, eat as much as you want from this list. Winter squash is not on this list due to their starch content. No offense intended to the winter squashes of the world, they are very healthy, but if you're not a potato, you didn't make the cut, sorry!

TIP: Eat only when hungry and just enough that you feel satisfied. You should feel comfortably full but not stuffed.

THE POTATO RESET
Guidelines at a Glance

UNLIMITED

POTATOES

Any variety such as red, yellow, gold, white, russet, sweet, purple, yams, etc. Eat until satisfied but not uncomfortably full.

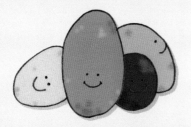

DRINKS

Water, unsweetened soda water and herbal tea. To flavor to your water try adding sliced cucumbers, fresh lemon or lime.

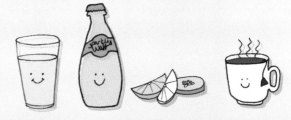

NON-STARCHY VEGETABLES

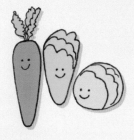

Artichoke	Cabbage	Kale	Rutabaga
Artichoke hearts	Carrots	Kohlrabi	Spinach
Arugula	Cauliflower	Leeks	Sprouts
Asparagus	Celery	Mushrooms	Summer Squash
Baby Corn	Collard Greens	Mustard Greens	Sugar Snap Peas
Bamboo Shoots	Cucumber	Okra	Swiss Chard
Bean Sprouts	Daikon	Onions	Tomato
Beets	Eggplant	Pea Pods	Turnips
Brussels Sprouts	Green Beans	Peppers	Water Chestnuts
Broccoli	Hearts of Palm	Radishes	Yard-Long Beans
Bok Choy	Jicama	Romaine	Zucchini

TIP: load up on the veggies to speed up weight loss!

LIMITED

Homemade sauces, fat-free condiments with the least amount of sugar & sodium, maple or date syrup (max 2 tbsp per day), unsweetened non-dairy milk, coffee, black tea, kombucha and green tea.

AVOID

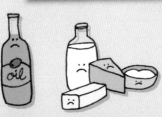

Oil, nuts, seeds, avocado, dairy products such as milk/butter/cheese/sour cream, eggs, meat, fish, processed sugar and artificial sweeteners.

Tips for Success

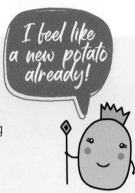

TOP TATER TIP! Always have leftover cooked/baked potatoes in the fridge! You can eat them cold in a pinch, or you can easily shred them into hash browns, make smashed potatoes or wedges, and reheat until crisp! See the batch cooking section on page 36 for more information how to batch cook.

I feel like a new potato already!

Journal Your Experience

In addition to writing out a list of goals, I encourage you to keep a journal of your Potato Reset experience. It doesn't have to be meticulously detailed; simply writing out a short summary of how your day went would be sufficient. Note any changes in your cravings, emotions, energy, or anything from your goals list that may be improving.

Control Your Environment

You can't always control what temptations may be lurking outside your home, but you can create a safe zone inside your home. Create a "safe zone" in your fridge and pantry (or a drawer/cupboard). Better yet, if you can pull it off, make your entire kitchen free of non-potato-cleanse foods except for ONE area that only your family has access to (locked perhaps?).

Get Organized

Organize your dry spices and your fridge so that it's easy for you to throw together something tasty. I have easy access to all my spices, plus I have an area of the fridge just for me: where I keep my lemons, homemade sauces, and mustard. Keep tempting foods out of your house if possible or in an area that you can't access.

Do I Need to Weigh My Potatoes?

Not on a regular basis, no. The only reason I'd ever suggest weighing your potatoes is so you know how many pounds you need to purchase. And it is kind of fun to brag to family and friends that you ate so many pounds of potatoes and lost weight! I weighed my potatoes a couple of times because everyone wanted to know how much I ate in a day, which turned out to be approximately 4 lbs.

Do I Need to Count Calories?

Definitely not. One of the primary purposes of this way of eating is to learn to trust your body again (and for your body to trust you!). If you have a history of calorie-counting and this idea gives you stress, please consider weaning yourself off gradually. You will be eating one of the most satisfying foods on the planet—full of minerals and vitamins. It's very difficult to overeat on potatoes. Eat until satisfied but not uncomfortably full.

Go Easy on the Sauces

Stick with fat-free, vegan sauces—preferably low-sodium and homemade. Avoid drenching your potatoes in sauce, especially store-bought sauces. It's best to dip your potatoes into the sauce or dip your fork into the sauce first, rather than pouring it all over your potatoes. Sauces add calories that are not filling plus they can overstimulate your taste buds, increase appetite, and potentially cause you to eat beyond satiation.

Dining Out

Look up menus online, or call and ask what they have available. A baked potato without oil, butter, or salt is ideal. If it's a social function where you don't have a choice eat before you go and order a garden salad without dressing. Bring your own dressing or ask for mustard, balsamic vinegar, and lemon or lime to whip up your own dressing. Remind yourself that you're here for the people and not the food.

Travel Tips

Traveling by Air

At the airport, there are many temptations of fast food and junky snacks that can suddenly make your potatoes seem boring. I traveled a few times while potato dieting and baked baby potatoes are hands down my favorite little travel gems. If you can actually make oven-baked potato chips and manage to pack them without eating them first, they make an excellent travel companion, as well. Pack a really tasty sauce in a small leak-proof container – as long as it does not exceed the allowed size for liquids.

Traveling by Car

The best part about traveling by car is that you have the ability to pack a cooler. I suggest bringing Potato Salad, some oil-free baked chips, baked potatoes, fresh cut veggies, your favorite reset friendly sauce and something fun to drink, such as homemade unsweetened iced tea, soda water with lemon, or a bottle of kombucha. If your destination is a hotel room, bring a rice cooker and a George Foreman grill if you can, or try to get a hotel room with a microwave.

Accommodations with a Kitchen

The best case scenario is to find accommodations with a kitchen. Airbnb are great as many come equipped with a full kitchen. Some hotels have kitchenettes with a microwave, sink and mini-fridge.

When in Doubt, Eat Whole Plant Foods

Travel doesn't always go as planned. Be mentally prepared to allow for other foods in a pinch. Also, know that it is okay to skip a meal if you can't find something suitable. If you must "cheat" on the Potato Reset, you are better off eating fruit or other whole plant foods instead of something junky. Here's some meal ideas for when you're in a sticky situation:

- **Baked Potato:** The ideal situation would be a baked potato and a garden salad with mustard or balsamic vinegar.

- **Oatmeal:** When flying, I always like to pack quick oats and sometimes dried fruit. You can find a coffee shop just about anywhere; just ask for hot water plus an extra cup. Bam, you have oatmeal! I never travel without oats.

- **Rice & Veggies:** I've had success at several Asian restaurants by asking if they are able to make plain steamed rice and plain steamed veggies without salt or oil. Add a little hot sauce or Thai chili sauce if needed.

Potato Cuts

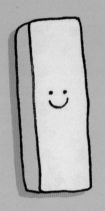
STEAK FRY

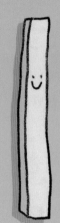
SKINNY FRY

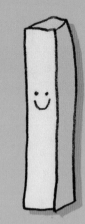
NORMAL FRY

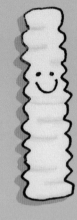
CRINKLE FRY

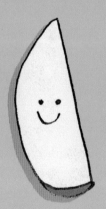
WEDGE

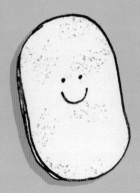
CHIP

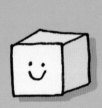
CUBED

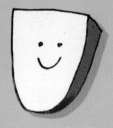
QUARTERED

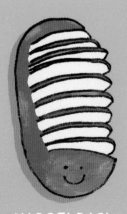
HASSELBACK

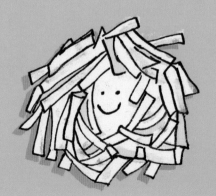
SHREDDED

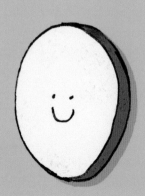
ROUNDS

Veggie Cuts

SLICED

CUBED

DICED

MINCED

CHOPPED

JULIENNE

Helpful Kitchen Tools

ALL YOU REALLY NEED ARE THE BASICS: soup pots, vegetable scrubber, baking sheets, potato masher, a sharp knife, cutting board, oven and parchment paper. Please don't feel that you can't do this without fancy kitchen tools. Even if all you have is a microwave or a camping stove and soup pots: you can do this! Check your local second hand shops for small appliances such as indoor electric grills like the George Foreman, waffle makers and toaster ovens. For links to all my favorite products go to **kit.com/jeannineelder**

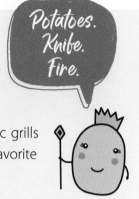

Potatoes. Knife. Fire.

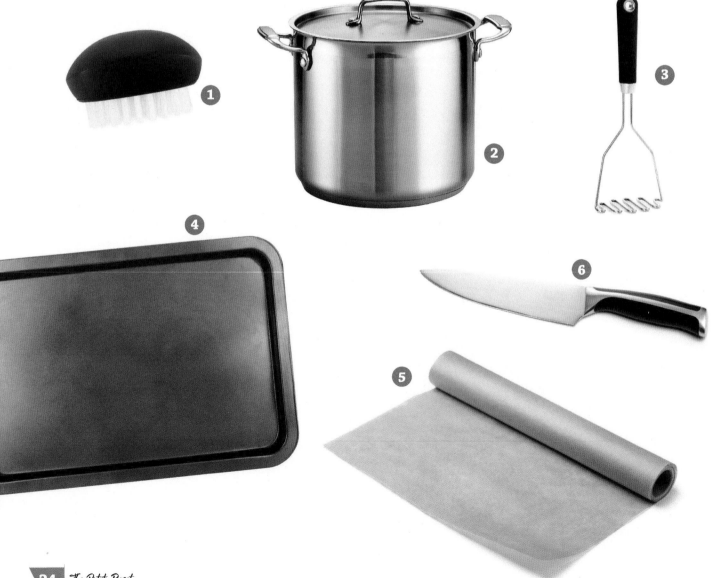

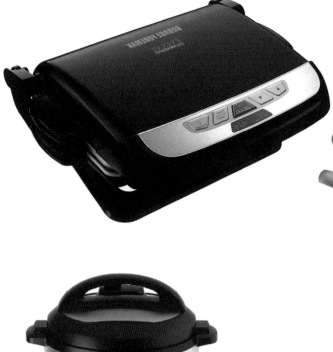

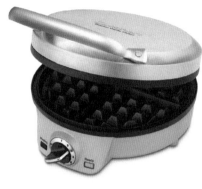

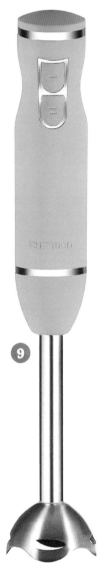

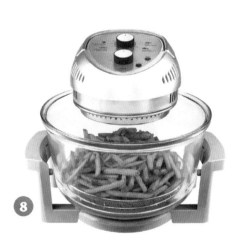

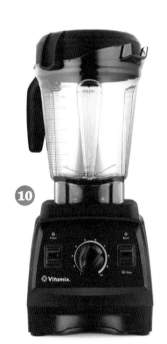

MUST HAVES:
1. Vegetable Scrubber
2. Soup Pots
3. Potato Masher
4. Baking Sheets
5. Parchment Paper
6. Sharp Knife

NICE TO HAVE:
7. George Foreman Grill, Waffle or Panini Maker
8. Air Fryer
9. Immersion Blender
10. High-Powered Blender
11. Pressure Cooker

LINKS TO ALL
PRODUCTS HERE
kit.com/jeannineelder

Meal Plan Guidelines

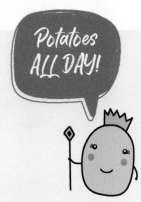

Potatoes ALL DAY!

THIS MEAL PLAN is to give you ideas on how to structure your meals. You don't have to follow it exactly. You may find yourself only hungry for two meals a day if you eat large meals like myself. Go with whatever works for you. Remember, eat when you are truly hungry and eat until satisfied – you should never feel uncomfortably full.

Preparing Breakfast

You won't see smoothies, toast, cereal and super quick breakfast ideas here. But I've picked out the quickest of the bunch. It literally takes me two minutes to shred a few leftover baked potatoes and throw it in the oven or on the George Foreman grill. I could honestly eat crispy hash browns every day! Another quick meal is Crispy Smashed Potatoes – slice a leftover baked potato in half and smash it down with a fork, bake it until crisp. Done! While my potatoes are cooking I get ready for my day.

Packing a Lunch

For this meal plan, I was mindful of those who have to pack their lunch for work or school. Five out of the seven days include portable meal ideas that are either okay to eat cold or can easily be reheated. You will see I chose soups, fresh-cut veggies, salad greens, and potato salad. If you don't have access to a microwave (or you don't like microwaves) just heat up your soup and steamed veggies at home and store in a thermos to keep it warm. Potatoes can always be eaten cold. It may be boring but this plan isn't meant to be exciting.

Dinners for Busy People

Some of the recipes can seem time consuming to those who literally have no time to spare. If this is you I suggest you make it a priority to batch cook at least once per week. One hour in the kitchen on a Sunday can set you up for the work week.

Fill your oven with baked potatoes, get a large pot full of diced potatoes boiling and in another pot cook up a hearty potato soup.

Once everything is cooled, store in airtight containers in the fridge. Recipes like Oven Baked Fries can be swapped out for wedges that you make from leftover baked potatoes. Simply take your cold baked potato, slice it into wedges, season and bake until crisp.

TIP: Always have a back-up plan when trying a new recipe. It can take a couple of attempts to master the perfect oven-baked fries, hash browns, and grilled potato cakes.

NOTE: It's better to have too many potatoes than not enough, you can always batch-cook potatoes before they go bad.

7 Day Meal Plan

	BREAKFAST	LUNCH	DINNER
1	French Toast Sticks Herbal tea	Creamy Potato Leek Soup Cold baked potato with Smoky Sweet Mustard Dip	Oven Baked Fries over a large leafy green salad House Dressing 2.0
2	Crispy Smashed Potatoes BBQ Sauce Steamed veggies	Creamy Potato Leek Soup Celery & carrot sticks with No-Honey Mustard Dip	Creamy Potato Leek Soup Potato Chips Steamed veggies & Unicorn Dust
3	Crispy Hash Browns BBQ Sauce	Potato Salad over a bowl of salad greens House Dressing 2.0	Pakoras Roasted Broccoli Smoky Sweet Mustard Dip
4	Crispy Grilled Potato Pancakes Marinara Sauce	Potato Salad over a bowl of salad greens House Dressing 2.0	Oven Baked Fries over a large leafy green salad House Dressing 2.0
5	Smoky Sweet Potato Rounds No-Honey Mustard Dip	Boiled Taters n' Dill Steamed veggies & Unicorn Dust	Veggie Soup Roasted Rosemary Garlic Potatoes
6	Broccoli Tots Unsweetened Ketchup	Veggie Soup Roasted Rosemary Garlic Potatoes (reheat leftovers)	Chili Cheeze Fries over a large bowl of romaine lettuce
7	Potato Rounds Amazing Cheeze Sauce	Broccoli Cheddar Soup Crispy Smashed Potatoes	Creamy Mashed Potatoes Golden Gravy

Grocery List

PRODUCE
- 10 lbs russet potatoes
- 5 lbs yellow potatoes
- 5 lbs red potatoes
- 4 medium sweet potatoes
- 3 or more servings of veggies for steaming
- leafy salad greens
- 2 lbs broccoli crowns
- 1 container of baby spinach
- 1 small head cauliflower
- 1 bunch celery
- 2 lbs carrots
- 1 small cabbage
- 1 bulb of garlic
- 1 bunch green onion
- 1 bunch leeks
- 2 small sweet onions
- 2-3 each lemons & limes

CONDIMENTS
- 2 small cans tomato paste
- 1 bottle of molasses
- 1 can fire roasted tomatoes
- 6.5 cups (52 oz) no-salt-added vegetable broth or vegetable bouillon
- 1 can diced tomatoes
- 1 jar strained tomatoes
- stone ground mustard
- dijon mustard
- maple syrup
- balsamic vinegar
- white vinegar (optional)
- Braggs Liquid Aminos or Coconut Aminos (optional)
- liquid smoke (optional)

SPICES
- potato starch
- nutritional yeast
- garlic powder
- onion powder
- smoked paprika
- cumin powder
- yellow curry powder
- garam masala
- tumeric
- Italian seasoning
- dried dill
- dried basil
- dried rosemary
- cayenne (optional)

Spice Up Your Taters!

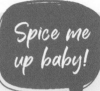
Spice me up baby!

IT'S EASY TO ADD FLAVOR to your potatoes without the oil, fat and salt you may be used to. There are many commercial spice blends available, but I find most to be filled with preservatives and salt. You are welcome to use salt, but use it sparingly and don't cook with it – instead, salt the top of your food just before you eat it so you won't need as much and you have more control of your sodium intake. Below are some store-bought options, and on the next page are some homemade spice blend recipes to spark your culinary creativity!

Spice Shopping Tips

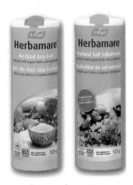

Salt Substitutes
Finding a reduced-salt or sodium-free salt substitute such as Herbamare is a great way to wean your palate off salt. Many of these are available in health food stores or online shops such as Amazon and Vitacost.

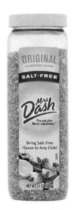
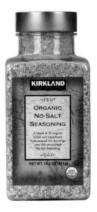

Salt-Free Seasoning Blends
Mrs. Dash Original and Kirkland's No-Salt Seasoning are similar in taste, in my opinion. Neither are my favorite, but I know a lot of people who love both. Benson's Table Tasty also has many flavors available and is by far my favorite, though not as easy to find.

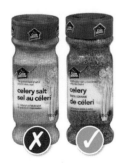

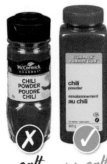
salt   no salt

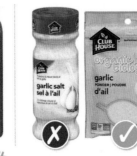

Read the Ingredients
Always check the ingredients list on every packaged product you purchase. Watch out for salt, sugar and oil! Recently, I was surprised to learn that some brands of vegetable bouillon cubes contain oil.

Spice Blend Recipes

THESE HOMEMADE blends are a great way to save money over store-bought spice blends. Other than the Salt Alternative, I have not specified how many servings you will get out of each spice blend because the amount you use will depend on how you are using it. Most of these blends last three or more batches of fries but if you're sprinkling a little into your hash browns it will last much longer. Typically, one baking sheet full of fries will need 2 teaspoons worth of spices.

Salt Substitute
¼   cup sea salt
2   tbsp dried parsley
½   tsp onion powder
½   tsp garlic powder
½   tsp oregano
½   tsp rosemary
½   tsp thyme
½   tsp sage
½   tsp basil
½   tsp celery seed
½   tsp marjoram
½   tsp dried kelp

Place all ingredients in a food processor or blender and blend until fine. Store in an airtight container. If your goal is to wean off salt, reduce amount of sea salt in each batch you make. 305mg of sodium per ¼ tsp servings – makes 92 servings.

Unicorn Dust
¼   cup nutritional yeast
1   tbsp garlic powder
1   tsp onion powder

Crush into a fine powder with a mortar & pestle or coffee grinder. Sprinkle on steamed veggies!

Simple Indian
1   tsp mild yellow curry powder
1   tsp onion powder

Indian
1   tsp garam masala
1   tsp mild yellow curry powder
½   tsp ground ginger
¼   tsp nutmeg
¼   tsp paprika
¼   tsp turmeric

Taco Seasoning
2   tsp chili powder
1   tsp cumin
1   tsp garlic powder
1   tsp onion powder
¼   tsp oregano

Spicy Cajun
2   tsp smoked paprika
1   tsp garlic powder
1   tsp onion powder
½   tsp black pepper
¼   tsp cayenne pepper

Ranch
1   tbsp dried parsley
1   tsp dried dill
1   tsp garlic powder
1   tsp onion powder

French
1   tbsp thyme
1   tsp garlic powder
½   tsp rosemary
½   tsp oregano
½   tsp Herbs de Provence

Caribbean
2   tsp allspice
1   tsp ground ginger
1   tsp garlic powder
1   tsp onion powder
½   tsp cinnamon
¼   tsp nutmeg
¼   tsp cloves

Mediterranean
1   tsp oregano
1   tsp rosemary
1   tsp thyme
1   tsp cardamom

BBQ
1   tbsp onion powder
1   tbsp smoked paprika
1   tsp chili powder
1   tsp Herbamare or other salt alternative
¼   tsp ground ginger
¼   tsp garlic powder
¼   tsp dried thyme
¼   tsp black pepper

Your Guide to Sauces

WHETHER YOU'RE INTO making homemade sauces or just want to keep it simple with store-bought, this guide to sauces will have you covered. Homemade is ideal but if you're not up for making homemade sauces or find yourself in a pinch, use this saucy shopping guide as a reference. In general you want to look for the lowest sugar and lowest sodium version you can find. The reason for this is that the potato reset is meant to reset your taste buds and calm the junk food cravings. Salt and sugar tend to stimulate the taste buds, we want to underwhelm the taste buds. We're also going to avoid anything with dairy and oil – both very calorically dense.

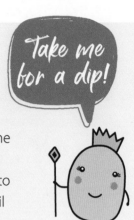

Take me for a dip!

🛒 Sauce Shopping Tips

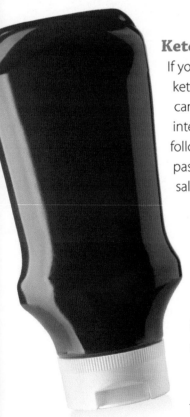

MY FAVORITE MUSTARD!

Ketchup

If your grocery store only has one type of ketchup, don't sweat it, just do the best you can. You can turn down the salty sugary intensity by diluting it with any of the following: water and no-salt-added tomato paste, strained tomatoes or blend with no-salt-added canned diced tomatoes.

BBQ Sauce

Woah! Hold on there partner, BBQ sauces are loaded with sodium! Most are around 250 mg per two table-spoons while compared to 160 mg for ketchup. So what's a BBQ sauce lover to do? Avoid high fructose corn syrup and go for the one with lowest sodium and sugar you can find. You can turn down the salty sugary intensity by diluting your BBQ sauce in some water and no-salt-added tomato paste.

Mustard

My go-to is Westbrae Natural's No Salt Added Stone Ground Mustard. You can have as much of it as you want as it's free of sugar and salt! If you find it too bland you can always mix half and half with regular salted stone ground mustard. If you prefer classic yellow mustard, go with the lowest sodium you can find. For a honey mustard substitute, mix 3 to 1 mustard and 100% pure maple syrup.

Maple Syrup

Look for 100% Pure Maple syrup, none of that imitation stuff (sorry Aunt Jemima). Another option is date syrup or home made date paste. This is only for using in sauce recipes and not intended as a dip on it's own as it can be very overstimulating and trigger cravings.

istockphoto.com

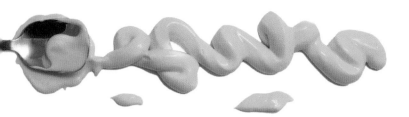

Vinegar

Have you ever had malt vinegar on french fries? Depending on where you grew up, it might sound odd but you never know, you just might like it. It's good to have on hand balsamic or apple cider vinegar for use in salad dressing recipes. Balsamic is sharp while apple cider vinegar is mild and slightly sour. Balsamic vinegar can be a lifesaver for someone with a sweet tooth or an aversion to veggies – roast some veggies in a good quality balsamic and the result is sweet and crunchy. If you can find a balsamic vinegar with 4% acidity, it's worth the extra money. Napa Valley Naturals Grand Reserve has 4% acidity and highly recommended by Chef AJ.

Soy Sauce

Soy sauce is very high in sodium and not to be used on it's own. I've only included it here because it's included in a couple of gravy recipes in this book, but is not required. Bragg's Liquid Amino's is my soy sauce of choice, it's lower in sodium than most soy sauces and it's Non-GMO. Alternatively you can use coconut aminos, reduced-sodium soy sauce or miso paste.

Hot Sauce

Many hot sauces are high in sodium, but if you're a hot sauce fan you know that a little goes a long way. If you are hot for hot sauce just cut it back a little. Or if you can, get your hands on some Trader Joe's Chili Pepper Sauce, go to town on it because it's sodium free. For me, spicy hot is out of the question, I always want something sweet after eating spicy food.

I FOUND THIS ONLINE BY GOOGLING 'NO SODIUM HOT SAUCE'

Salsa

Salsas are great because they are easy to find just about anywhere! I rarely come across salsas with added oil but always double check the ingredients. Just to be consistent with the plan, avoid salsas with beans and corn – which are both starches. Get the lowest sodium and lowest sugar version you can find. To dilute the saltiness of your salsa, mix a 1 to 1 ratio of salsa and no salt added diced or crushed tomatoes.

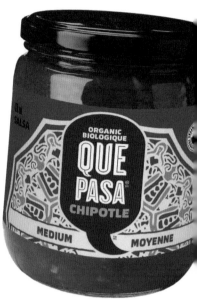

Creamy Sauces

Sorry, there's nothing I can personally recommend that meets the guidelines of the Potato Reset other than making your own. See Potato Ranch Dressing on page 34)

Pickled & Fermented Veggies

Add flavor and texture to your potatoes with dill pickles, banana peppers and sauerkraut. Just keep in mind most are high in sodium so keep it minimal.

Other

If your sauce is not on the list, check the ingredients: avoid if it has oil, dairy or any animal ingredients. Proceed with caution if it's high in sodium or sugar – be creative and think of ways to dilute it.

Tater Tip!

DIP BUT DON'T DRENCH! Place your store-bought sauce into a small dipping bowl to avoid overdoing it.

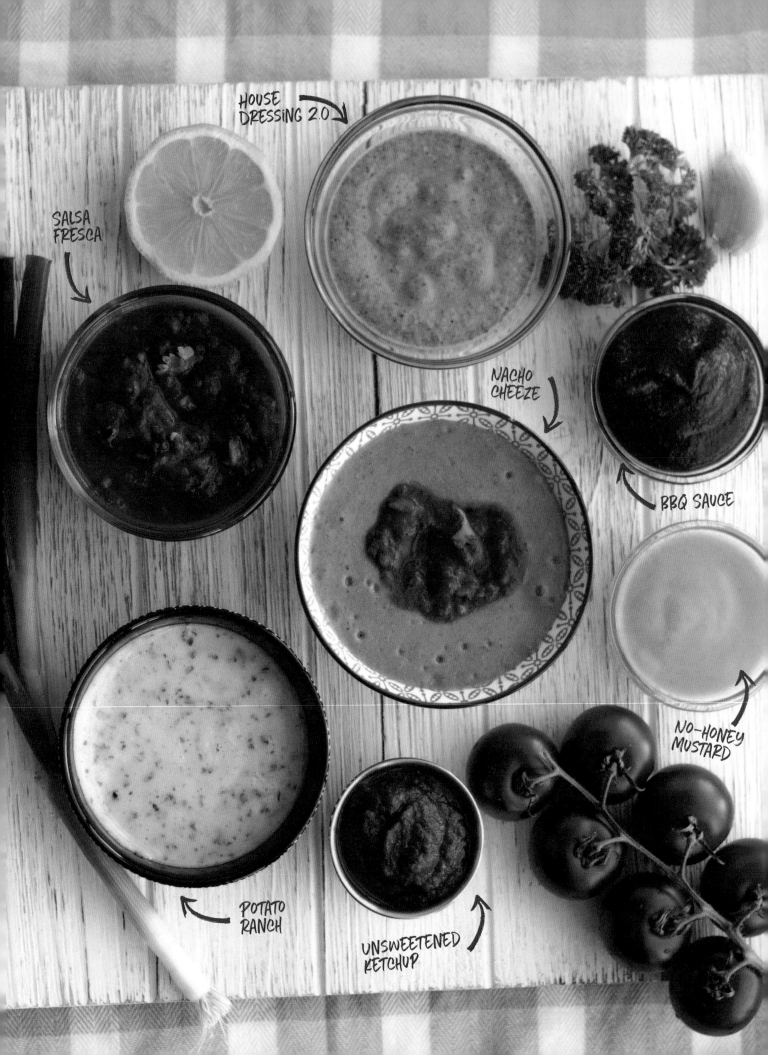

HOUSE DRESSING 2.0

SALSA FRESCA

NACHO CHEEZE

BBQ SAUCE

NO-HONEY MUSTARD

POTATO RANCH

UNSWEETENED KETCHUP

Homemade Sauces

Simple Salad Dressing

2   tbsp nutritional yeast

2   tbsp balsamic vinegar (4% acidity, if possible)

1   tbsp mustard

1   lemon or lime, juiced

1   tbsp maple syrup

1   tsp Bragg's Liquid Aminos or coconut aminos

Whisk together. Stores well in fridge for 3 days.

Chef AJ's House Dressing 2.0

2   tbsp reduced balsamic vinegar

2   tbsp lime juice

1   tbsp no-salt-added stone ground mustard

Chef AJ's easiest dressing; just stir together and enjoy on vegetables and salads. Find Chef AJ at: eatunprocessed.com

No-Honey Mustard Dip

2   tbsp dijon or stone ground mustard

1   tsp pure maple syrup

Stir together and enjoy! Feel free to experiment with different types of mustard.

Smoky Sweet Mustard Dip

2   tbsp mustard, any kind

1   tsp pure maple syrup

¼   tsp liquid smoke or smoked paprika

Stir together and enjoy! Once again, you can experiment with different types of mustard.

Unsweetened Ketchup

¼   cup strained tomatoes (no salt added)

1   tbsp white vinegar

½   tsp onion powder

½   tsp Italian seasoning

Stir until smooth. If you're just starting out and this tastes really bland to you, try adding a pinch of salt.

Curry Ketchup

2   6oz cans tomato paste

1   cup water

1   tsp onion powder

1   tbsp maple or date syrup

1   tbsp lemon juice

1   tbsp apple cider vinegar

1   tsp curry powder

Blend in a blender or whisk together until smooth.

Hot Sauce

1   roasted red bell pepper
(if you get this in a jar make sure oil-free)

1   tbsp rice vinegar or apple cider vinegar

1   clove garlic

¼   tsp chipotle powder

¼   tsp smoked paprika

¼   tsp onion powder

Blend in a blender until smooth.

Homemade Sauces

Marinara Sauce

1   14-oz can fire roasted tomatoes
1   tsp balsamic vinegar
1   tsp pure maple syrup
1   tsp Italian seasoning
¼   tsp liquid smoke, optional

Blend all ingredients in blender until smooth.

BBQ Sauce

¾   cup tomato paste (5.5 fl oz / 156 mL)
½   cup water
2   tbsp apple cider vinegar
1   tbsp maple or date syrup (optional)
1   tbsp molasses
1   tbsp liquid smoke
1   tbsp mustard
½   tsp garlic powder
½   tsp onion powder
½   tsp smoked paprika

Stir until smooth.

Potato Ranch

1   medium boiled potato
¼   cup unsweetened almond milk
2   tbsp lemon juice
1   tbsp apple cider vinegar
1   tsp onion powder
½   tsp garlic powder
1   tbsp dried parsley
1   tsp dried chives

Place all ingredients, except for the dried parsley and dried chives, in a blender and blend until smooth. Stir in the dried herbs and serve.

Salsa Fresca

2   14-oz cans of fire-roasted diced tomatoes
½   small organic sweet onion, chopped into quarters
2   cloves of garlic
1   jalapeno, seeded
1   tbsp cumin
½   cup fresh cilantro leaves, finely chopped
1   lime, juiced

Put all ingredients in the blender except the tomatoes. Blend on the lowest speed until everything is chopped well. Then, add the tomatoes and pulse a few times until the desired consistency is achieved.

Nacho Cheeze Sauce
BY HIGH CARB HANNAH

2   small red potatoes, quartered
½   small white onion, peeled
¼   cup of the potato cooking water
½   red bell pepper
½   cup nutritional yeast
1   tsp onion powder
1   tsp garlic powder
2   tbsp salsa
1   tbsp hot sauce (optional)
    salt to taste (optional)

Add potatoes and onion to a pot and cover with water. Bring to a boil, reduce heat to simmer and cook until soft. With a slotted spoon remove onion and potatoes from water and transfer to a blender. Add red pepper, nutritional yeast, garlic powder, onion powder, salsa, hot sauce and ¼ cup of the cooking water. Blend until smooth. Add water if needed. More of Hannah's recipes: *rawtillwhenever.com*

Amazing Vegan Cheeze Sauce
BY CHUCK UNDERWOOD

3   medium Yukon gold potatoes

2-3 large carrots

½   cup potato water

¼   cup nutritional yeast

2   tbsp nutritional yeast (in addition to above)

2   tbsp lemon juice

1   tsp apple cider vinegar

1   tsp salt (optional)

½   tsp onion powder

½   tsp garlic powder

½   tsp brown mustard

⅛   tsp turmeric

Wash and scrub both potatoes and carrots, peel if desired and chop into uniform pieces and boil for 10 minutes. Let rest for 5 minutes and then with a slotted spoon, transfer the veggies to your blender. Add 1/2 a cup of the potato water and pulse to mix then add remaining ingredients and blend until smooth. More of Chuck's amazing recipes: brandnewvegan.com

McDougall's Golden Gravy (modified)

1½ cups no-salt-added vegetable broth

½   cup water

½   tbsp Bragg's Liquid Aminos, coconut aminos or low sodium soy sauce

1   tsp onion powder

2   tbsp potato starch

In a small saucepan, whisk together the broth, water, aminos/soy sauce, potato starch and onion powder. Bring to a boil. Cook and stir continuously until thickened. Adapted from mcdougall.com

Creamy Mushroom Gravy

½   medium yellow or white potato, quartered or 1/2 cup potadough

1   cup no-salt-added vegetable broth

1   tbsp nutritional yeast

½   tbsp Bragg's Liquid Aminos, coconut aminos or low sodium soy sauce (optional)

¼   tsp onion powder

½   tsp garlic, minced

6   brown mushrooms, chopped

2   tbsp Italian seasoning

½   cup unsweetened non-dairy milk

If using a fresh potato, cover with water in a small pot and boil until soft, drain and set aside.

In a skillet, whisk together broth, nutritional yeast, onion powder, garlic and optional liquid aminos. Bring to a boil, then add mushrooms and Italian seasoning. Reduce heat to medium and simmer, stirring a few times, until the mushrooms are soft.

Place non-dairy milk, potato and mushroom mixture in a blender. Blend until smooth.

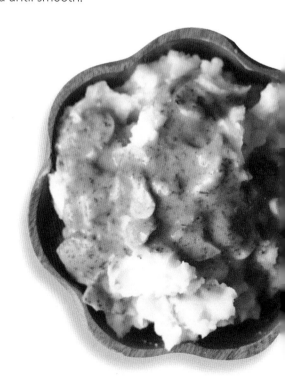

Batch Cooking

THE #1 KEY TO SUCCESS on this plan is to always have potatoes on hand, at least 5 pounds of potatoes in the pantry and cooked potatoes in the fridge. Having pre-cooked potatoes in the fridge ensures you will always have something ready to eat, and it will provide a base for many of the recipes in this book. Batch cooking also saves time and will help prevent you from eating off-plan foods . I recommend always having a batch of potadough, boiled or pressure cooker potatoes, baked potatoes, a homemade sauce, and if it's the right time of year, a batch of soup. Feel free to double up on these batch-cooking recipes.

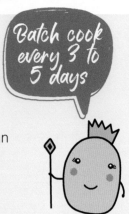

Batch cook every 3 to 5 days

Potadough

4   medium russet potatoes
2   tbsp no-salt-added vegetable
    broth or potato water

Wash, peel and cut your potatoes into quarters. Place in a stock pot and cover with water. Cook over high heat to bring water to a boil and continue cooking until fork tender. Watch that the water does not boil over; reduce heat if necessary.

Carefully drain, reserve some of the water if you're not using vegetable broth. Add the broth or potato water to the potatoes and mash with a handheld masher until you achieve a doughy consistency.

Do not use an immersion blender to mash as it will come out too gluey.

Stores in an airtight container in the fridge for 3 days.

FREEZE: Place on a parchment lined baking sheet in separate portion-size piles. Let freeze for 4 hours before transferring to a freezer bag. You can do this with mashed potatoes as well.

POTAYDOUGH CREATIONS:
- **Potato Crust Pizza**
- **Stuffed Potato Cakes**
- **Grilled Potato Cakes**

Baked Potatoes

Grab enough potatoes to fill at least one baking sheet, any kind: red, yellow, white or russets.

Preheat oven to 420°F. Wash potatoes and remove eyes or damaged spots from the potatoes.
Pierce each potato in two spots with a fork or knife. Place on baking sheet or directly on rack.

Bake for 45 - 60 minutes or until soft. This will depend on the size of your potato. If you are baking russets be sure to check on them around 40 minutes – I find if these are overcooked the skins become too tough. You want the potatoes to be just cooked enough so that they are soft but not too much that they dry out.

Eat a few now if you wish, and let the rest cool before storing in an airtight container in the fridge for up to five days. I usually eat mine up before three days.

BAKE POTATO CREATIONS:
- **Smashed potatoes**
- **Hash browns**
- **Frozen Shredded Hash Browns (next page)**
- **Broccoli Tots**
- **Wedges: slice into wedges and broil until crisp**
- **On-the-go cold snack**

Frozen Shredded Hash Browns

8 medium leftover cold baked potatoes

Shred the potatoes, using a hand held grater, into a large mixing bowl. Divide into 3 to 5 equal parts, depending on how much you need per meal, and place into freezer bags or airtight food storage containers.

Avoid pressing into one big clump, instead, place in storage device loosely but also don't leave room for air. Store in freezer for up to a month. When you're ready to cook, let the hash browns defrost at room temperature for 10-15 minutes or put them in the fridge the night before.

Boiled Potatoes

Enough potatoes to fill half of a large pot.
Any kind: Red, yellow, white or russets.

Wash potatoes, peel if desired and remove eyes or damaged spots. Cut into quarters or cubes, depending on preference.

Place potatoes in pot and fill with just enough water to cover potatoes. Bring to a gentle boil and continue cooking until potatoes are fork tender.

Drain and let cool before storing in an airtight container. Keeps well in the fridge for up to five days.

BOILED POTATO CREATIONS:
- **Potato salad**
- **Bake in the oven at 420°F until crisp**
- **Reheat in an air fryer or George Foreman grill until crisp**
- **Add on top of large green salad**

Pressure Cooker Potatoes

Enough potatoes to almost fill your pressure cooker.
Any kind: Red, yellow, white or russets.

1 cup water

Wash potatoes, peel if desired and remove eyes or damaged spots. Leave as they are, uncut, or if desired cut into quarters or cubes, depending on preference.

If you have wire rack that came with your pressure cooker, place it in the bottom. If not, don't worry, it still works without it. Add water then potatoes. Set to manual for 10 minutes, vent set to seal. Let pressure cooker release naturally.

Let cool before storing in an airtight container. Keeps well in the fridge for up to five days.

PRESSURE COOKER POTATO CREATIONS:
- **Hash browns**
- **Potato salad**
- **Smashed potatoes**
- **Eat as is: they are delicious cold!**

Frozen French Fries

4 medium russet potatoes

You will need two large soup pots, one for boiling and one for chilling. Fill half of one pot with ice water, along with ice cubes. Wash potatoes and slice into steak fries, wedges or normal fry cut. Place in large stock pot and cover with water. Bring to a boil and let cook for 2 minutes.

Drain from boiling water and immediately pour fries into ice bath. Let chill in ice bath for 5 minutes.

Drain fries from ice bath, pat dry on clean kitchen towels. Spread fries out on 2 parchment lined baking sheets. Let freeze for 6 hours or overnight.

Transfer frozen fries to zip-top freezer bags. Store for up to 6 months. See Oven Baked Fries recipe for cooking instructions.

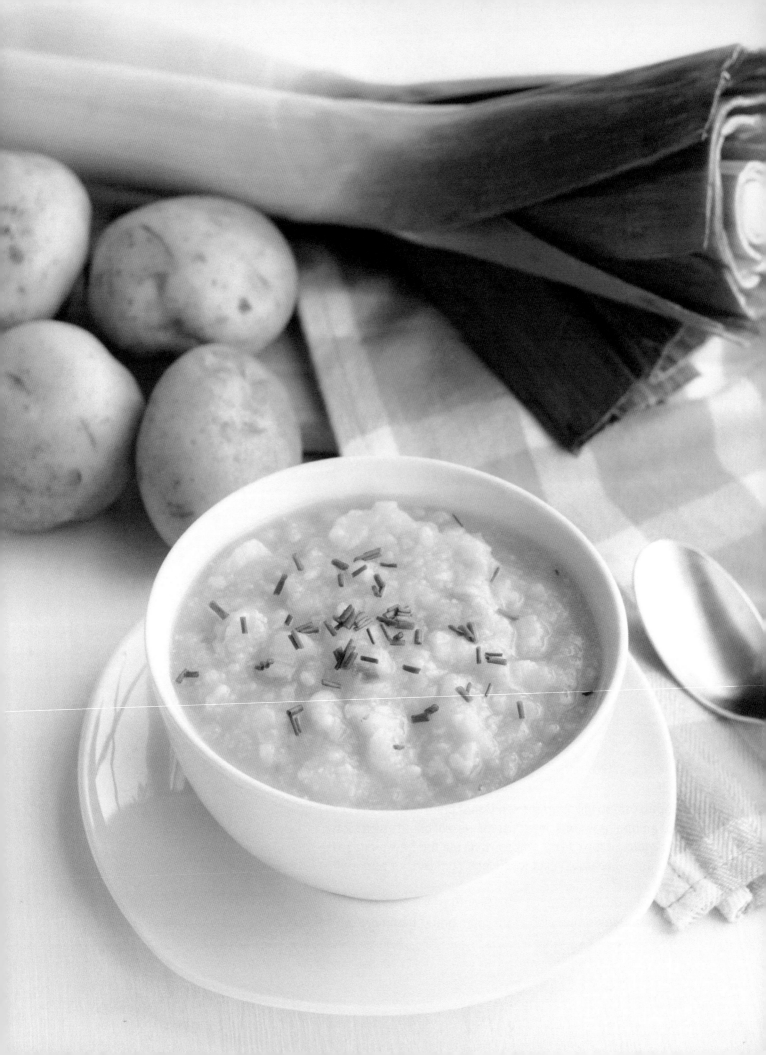

Creamy Potato Leek Soup

PREP TIME: 10 minutes | **COOK TIME:** 30 minutes | **SERVES:** 3-6

Ingredients

- 3 pounds potatoes, cubed
- 2 cups cauliflower, chopped
- 1 bunch leeks, chopped
- 1 stalk celery, chopped
- 1 clove garlic, minced
- 2 cups no-salt-added vegetable broth
- 1 tsp dried rosemary
- ground black pepper, to taste

Good With

A large leafy green salad

Method

Line a large pot with 1/4" of water; bring to a slight boil, then add garlic, leeks and celery. Reduce heat to medium and sauté until soft; stir often.

Add rosemary, cauliflower, potatoes and vegetable broth. Stir. Then, add enough water to cover everything – all potatoes and veggies should be submerged in liquid. Bring to a boil, then let simmer for 20 minutes or until potatoes are soft.

To make it creamy, you can either partially blend with an immersion blender or blend half the soup in a blender – it will be very hot, please make sure that the blender lid is tightly closed, then add the blended portion back into soup mixture.

Add ground black pepper to taste.

NO LEEKS? Try a variation of this with one bunch finely chopped green onions, or for a completely different flavor try it with a few carrots.

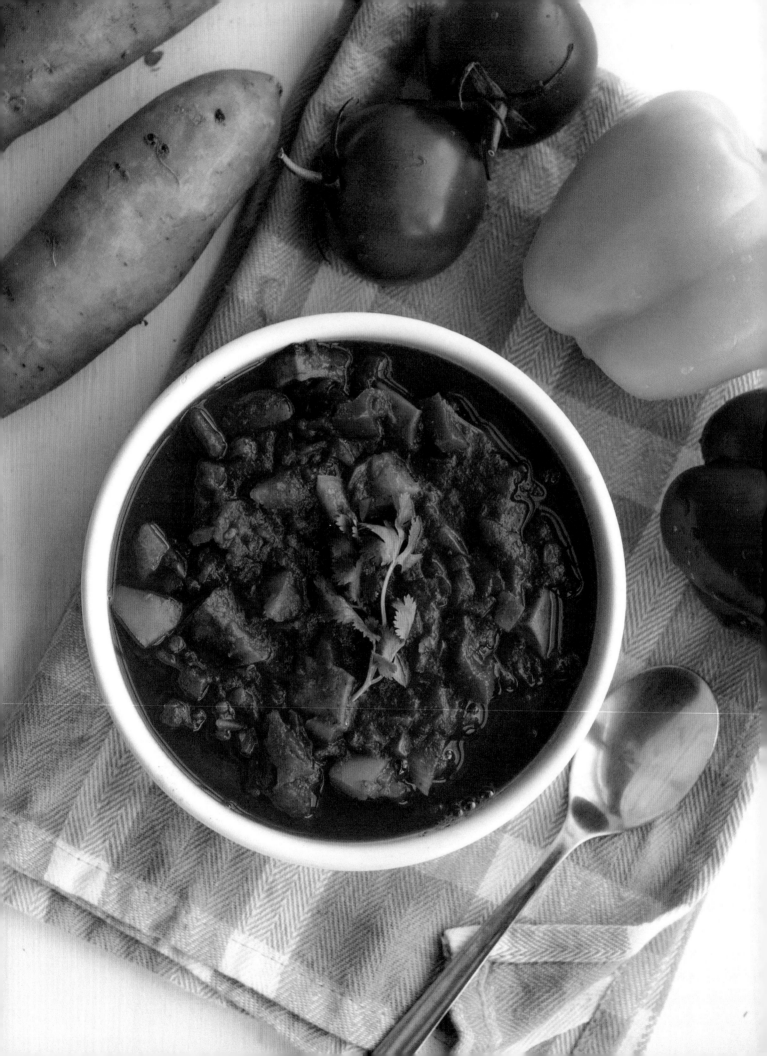

Sweet Potato Chili

PREP TIME: 10 minutes | **COOK TIME:** 45 minutes | **SERVES:** 2-3

Ingredients

- 2 medium sweet potatoes
- 1 tbsp chili powder
- 2 tsp ground cinnamon
- 1 tbsp ground cumin
- 1 tsp smoked paprika
- 1 medium yellow onion, chopped
- 1 red bell pepper, chopped
- 1 yellow bell pepper, chopped
- 1 large can of diced no-salt-added tomatoes
- ½ cup cilantro, finely chopped
- 1 cup no-salt-added vegetable broth

Good With

A large leafy green salad

Method

Preheat the oven to 350ºF. Line a baking sheet with parchment paper. Peel and cube the sweet potatoes. In a large bowl, toss with a pinch each of the chili powder, cinnamon, cumin and paprika. Spread out in an even layer on the baking sheet and roast in the oven for 35 to 40 minutes.

While the sweet potatoes are roasting, bring 1/4 cup of water to a gentle boil in a soup pot, sauté the onion and bell peppers until soft – about 3 minutes. Add vegetable broth and remaining chili powder, cinnamon, cumin and paprika. Cook over a low heat for 10 minutes, stirring often.

Add the diced tomatoes and simmer for 30 minutes. Stir in the sweet potatoes and cilantro leaves, serve.

VARIATION: For more traditional chili flavor, omit the cinnamon and add 1 tsp each garlic powder and ground cumin.

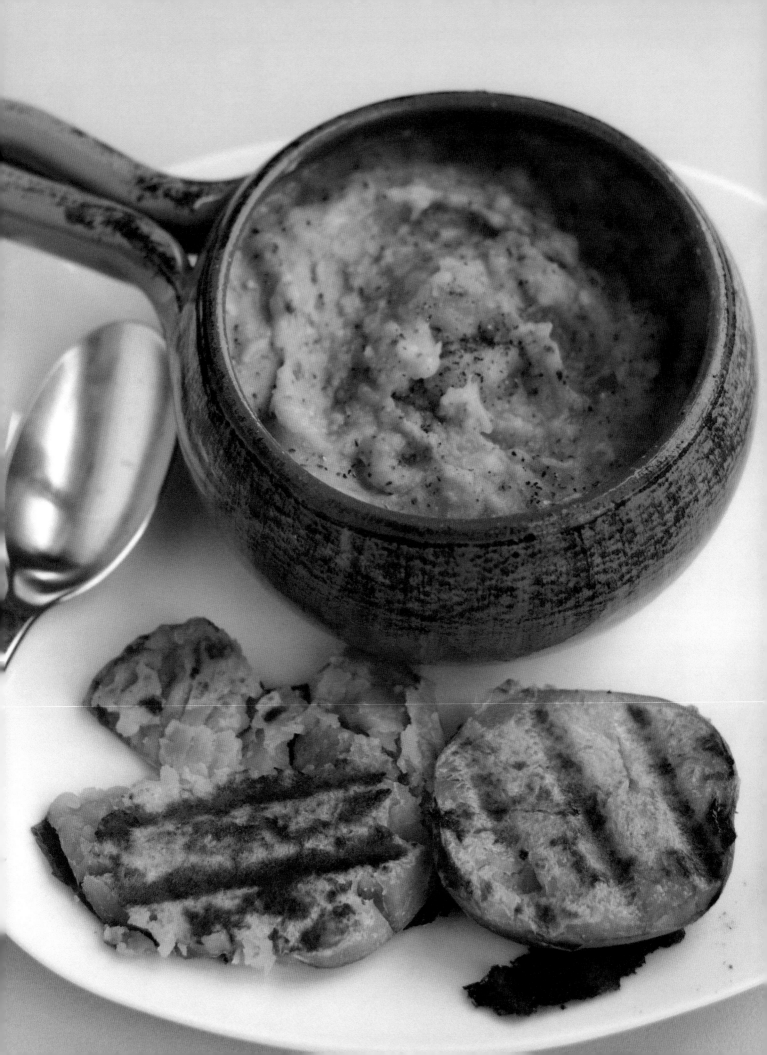

Broccoli Cheddar Soup

PREP TIME: 5 minutes | **COOK TIME:** 30 minutes | **SERVES:** 2-3

Ingredients

- 4 medium russet potatoes, peeled and cubed
- 4 cups broccoli, chopped
- ½ cup nutritional yeast
- 6 cups water (see note)
- 2 tsp Better Than Bouillon (or sub 2 cups of the water for 2 cups no-salt-added vegetable broth)
- 2 tsp garlic powder

Good With

Smashed Potatoes

Method

In a saucepan, cover potatoes with 3 cups water. Bring to a boil, reduce heat to a simmer and cover. Cook until soft (about 10 minutes).

Next, add in your broccoli, nutritional yeast, bouillon, remaining water and garlic powder. Cover and cook until broccoli is tender (about 5 minutes)

Take half your soup and blend in a blender until smooth. You can also use an immersion blender just make sure you don't blend everything completely, it's better if there are some chunks in it.

NOTE: I like mine super thick, so I use only 5 cups of total liquid by omitting one cup of water.

RECIPE PROVIDED BY HIGH CARB HANNAH
You can find this and many more delicious plant based recipes here: plantmealplanner.co and youtube.com/highcarbhannah

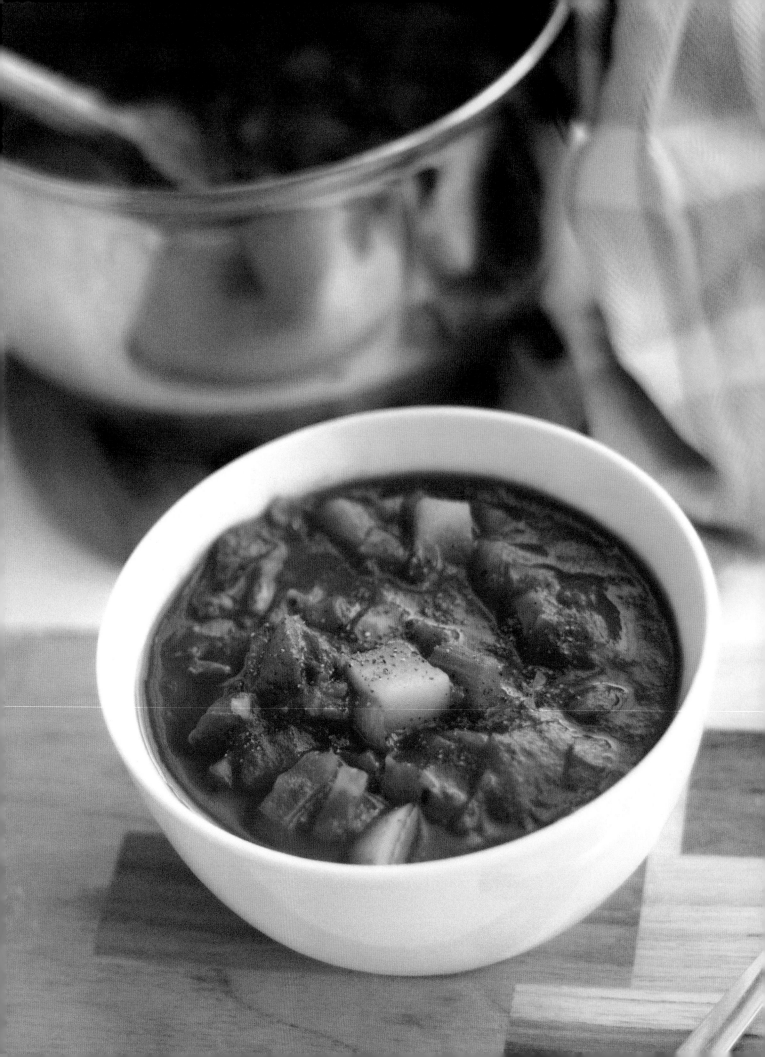

Hearty Veggie Soup

PREP TIME: 10 minutes | **COOK TIME:** 40 minutes | **SERVES:** 2-3

Ingredients

- 3 medium potatoes, peeled and cubed
- 1 28-oz can no salt added diced tomatoes
- 1 small can no-salt-added tomato paste
- 2 cups no-salt-added vegetable broth
- 1 cup water
- 1 small yellow onion, diced
- 2 stalks celery, diced
- 1 cup cabbage, chopped
- 1 tsp garlic powder
- 1 tsp dried basil

Good With

Oven Baked Fries or Crispy Potato Cakes

Method

Add a thin layer of water to a large soup pot. Water sauté the onions, celery and cabbage over medium heat, until onions are soft and translucent.

While the veggies are cooking, in a medium mixing bowl whisk the tomato paste, garlic powder and water.

Add the potatoes and diced tomatoes to the soup pot then pour in the tomato paste mixture and vegetable broth. Stir in the dried basil. Cover and simmer for 30 minutes or until potatoes are fork tender.

VARIATION: Swap out the cabbage for kale or spinach to use up what you might have in the fridge. Feel free to add in other veggies that you want to use up such as bell peppers and zucchini.

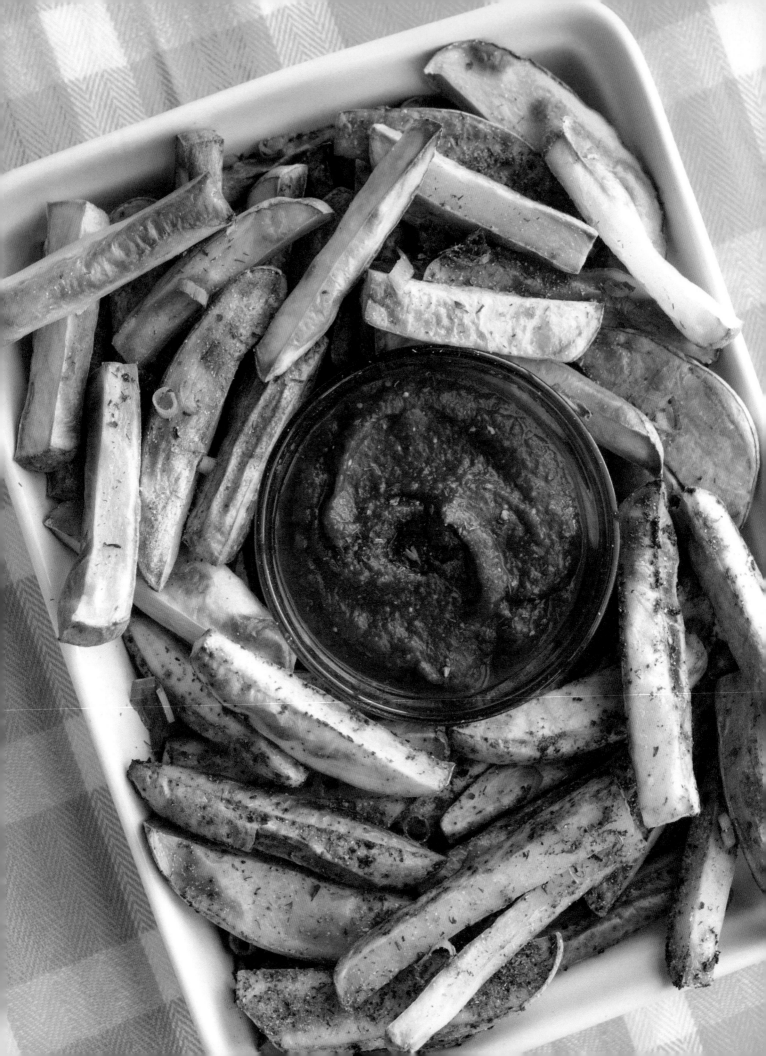

Oven Baked Fries

PREP TIME: 10 minutes | **COOK TIME:** 45 minutes | **SERVES:** 1-2

Ingredients

- 4 medium potatoes
- 2 tsp spices of choice, see examples below

CURRY FRIES
- 1 tsp onion powder
- 1 tsp curry powder

MEXI FRIES
- 1 tsp chili powder
- ½ tsp garlic powder
- ½ tsp onion powder

SOUR CREAM & ONION
- 1 tbsp apple cider vinegar (let sit for 15 minutes, drain excess vinegar then toss with spices)
- 1 tsp onion powder
- 1 tsp dried dill

Good With

Lettuce wraps & your favorite dip

Method

Preheat oven to 420°F. Line a baking sheet with parchment paper. Wash potatoes thoroughly and cut off any damaged spots, green skin or eyes.

Cut into steak fries. Choose a spice combo and in a large bowl mix with fries until well coated. Transfer to a the parchment-lined baking sheet. Avoid dumping excess spices onto the parchment as loose spices tend to burn.

Bake for 30 - 45 minutes until desired crispiness. Flip after 20 minutes. Cooking time varies oven to oven, keep a close eye after 30 minutes.

TIP: If you find that your fries are coming out hard on the inside and well done on the outside, reduce your oven temperature and cook for longer. Alternatively, steam or boil your fries for 10 minutes prior to baking.

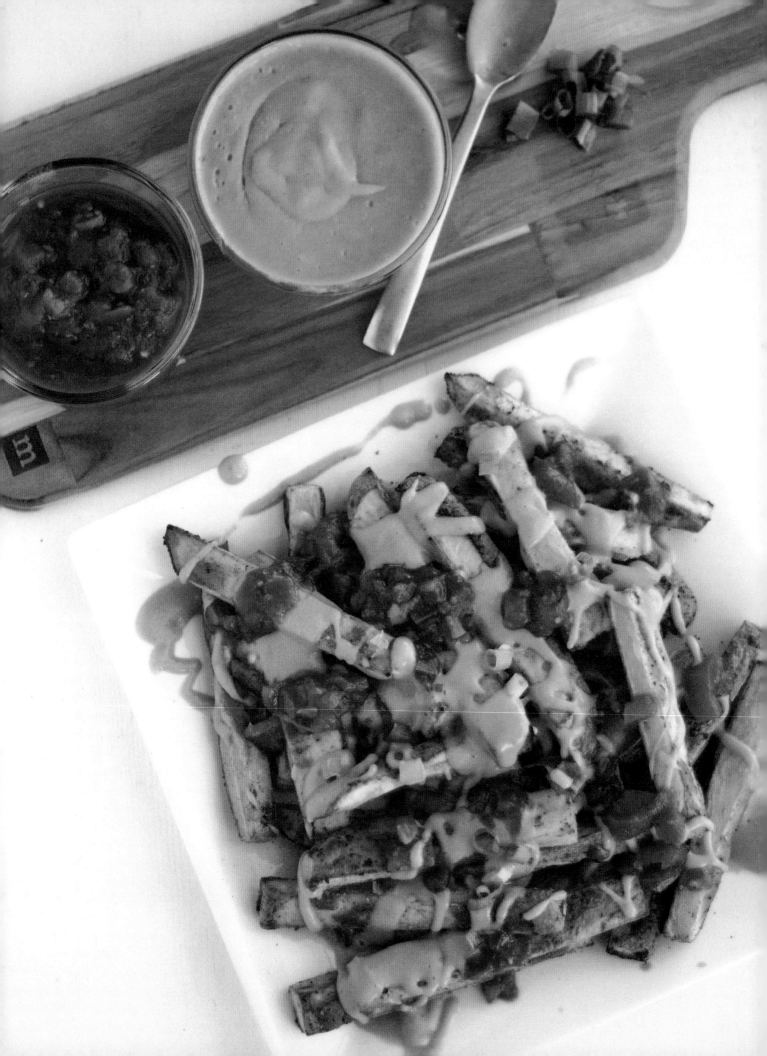

Chili Cheeze Fries

PREP TIME: 10 minutes | **COOK TIME: 40 minutes** | **SERVES: 1-2**

Ingredients

- 4 medium potatoes
- ½ tsp chili Powder
- ½ tsp garlic powder
- ½ tsp onion powder
- ¼ tsp cumin
- ¼ tsp oregano
- 1 green onion, chopped
- 1 cup crisp romaine lettuce, shredded
- 1 small tomato, diced

QUESO SAUCE

- 1 medium potato, quartered
- ½ small red onion
- ⅓ cup nutritional yeast
- 1 tsp garlic powder
- 1 tsp chili powder
- ¼ tsp cumin
- ⅓ cup salsa

Method

Preheat oven to 420°F. Line a baking sheet with parchment paper. Wash potatoes thoroughly and cut off any damaged spots, green skin or eyes.

Cut into thick strips. In a large bowl, toss strips with chili powder, garlic powder, onion powder, cumin and oregano. Transfer to a parchment-lined baking sheet. Avoid dumping excess spices onto the parchment as loose spices tend to burn.

Bake for 20 minutes, flip and bake for another 10 or until desired crispiness.

While the fries are baking: add a quartered medium potato to a small pot with water and boil until tender. Carefully transfer the boiled potato to a blender with a slotted spoon, reserve potato water. Then add onion, ¼ cup of the potato water, nutritional yeast, garlic powder, chili powder, cumin and salsa. Blend until smooth. Careful, it's hot, please make sure your blender lid is secure!

Plate fries and top with lettuce, queso sauce, green onion and diced tomato. Enjoy!

NOTE: Feel free to use any of the cheeze sauces from this book.

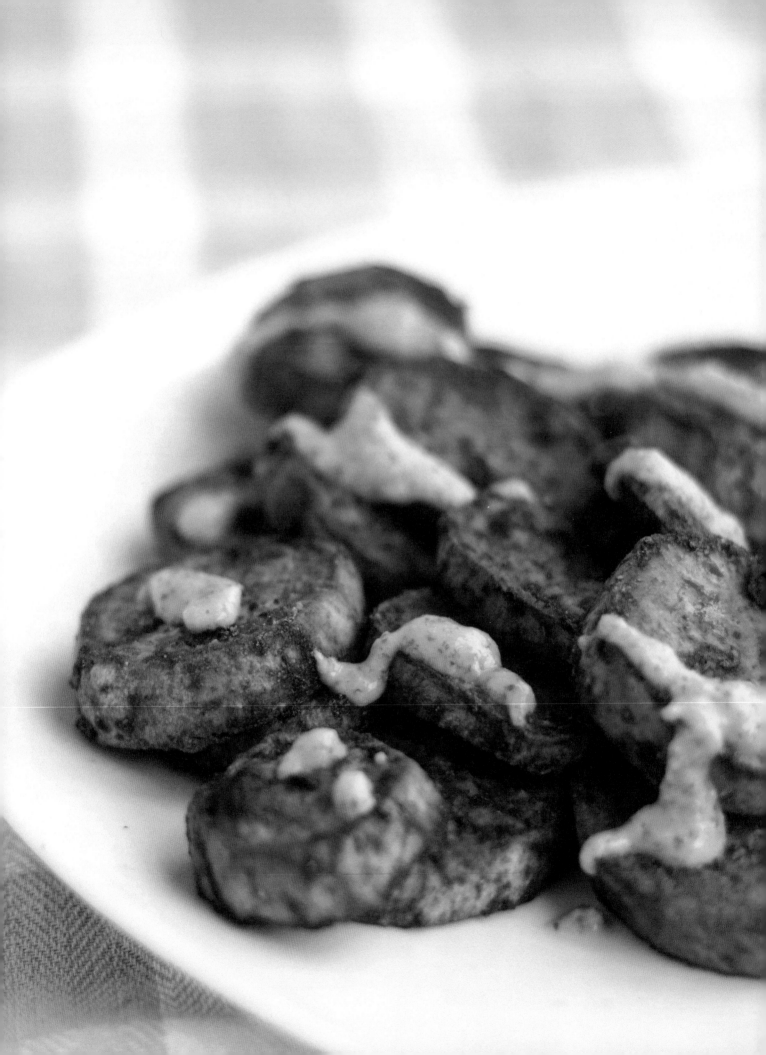

Smoky Sweet Potato Rounds

PREP TIME: 5 minutes | **COOK TIME:** 50 minutes | **SERVES:** 1

Ingredients

- 2 medium sweet potatoes
- 1 tbsp balsamic vinegar
- 1 tbsp pure maple syrup
- 1 tsp garlic powder
- ½ tsp dijon mustard
- ½ tsp smoked paprika
- ½ tsp liquid smoke (optional)

Good With

Smoky Sweet Mustard Dip

Method

Preheat oven to 375°F. Line a large baking sheet with parchment paper.

Wash and peel the sweet potatoes and cut into ¼" rounds . In a large bowl whisk together balsamic vinegar, maple syrup, dijon mustard, garlic powder, smoked paprika and liquid smoke. Place the rounds into the bowl and hand toss until well coated.

Spread wedges on parchment lined baking sheet and bake for 25 minutes, flip, bake for another 25 until they are lightly browned and slightly caramelized. Serve and enjoy!

VARIATION: swap out the maple syrup for extra mustard and balsamic vinegar for a more savory flavor.

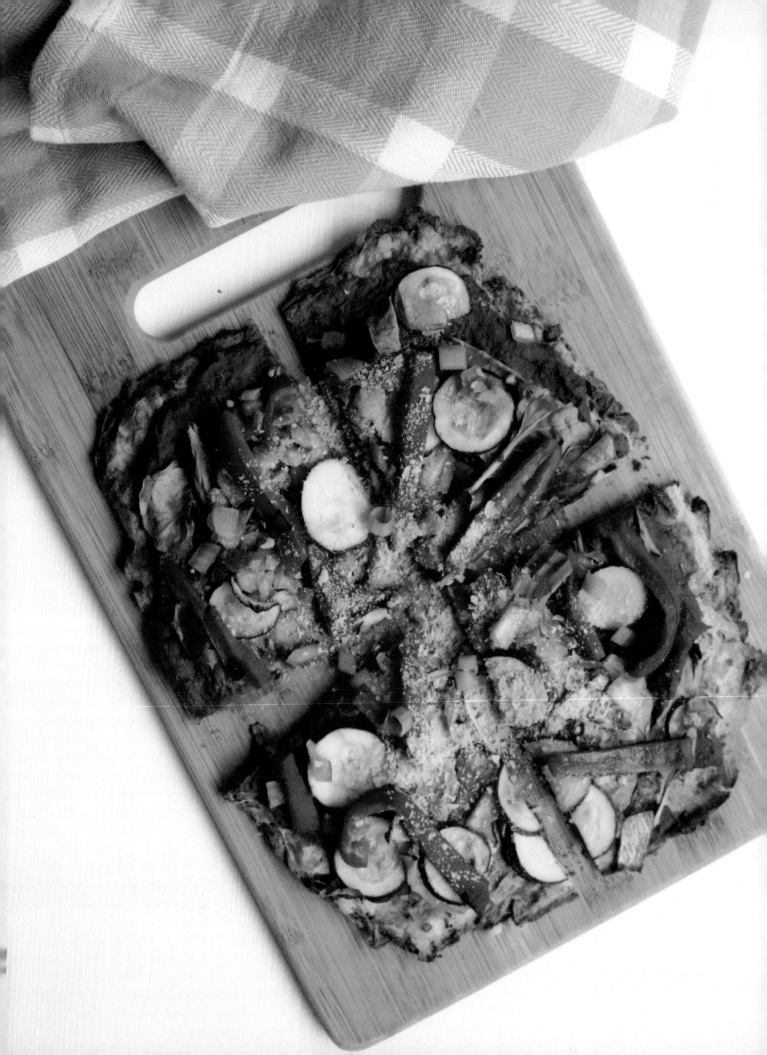

Potato Crust Pizza

PREP TIME: 10 minutes | **COOK TIME:** 40-50 minutes | **SERVES:** 1

Ingredients

CRUST

2-3 cups potadough

PIZZA SAUCE

2 small cans tomato paste (approx 12 oz total)

1 tsp garlic powder

1 tsp dried oregano

1 tsp dried basil

TOPPINGS

½ a small yellow or red onion, diced

4 mushrooms, sliced

1 bell pepper, thinly sliced

2 handfuls baby spinach

¼ cup nutritional yeast (optional)

Good With

Large leafy green salad

Method

Preheat oven to 420°F. Line baking sheet with parchment paper.

Place dough on the parchment-lined baking sheet to create a pizza crust shape, press down with your fingers until it's no more than ¼" thick. Bake for 30 minutes or longer, until just starting to turn golden brown. There shouldn't be any mushy spots.

Meanwhile, in a non stick skillet over medium-high heat, water sauté the onions, garlic, mushrooms and bell pepper until softened. Remove from heat and set aside.

In a small mixing bowl stir together tomato paste, garlic powder, onion powder, oregano and basil. Set aside.

Remove pizza from the oven, keeping on baking sheet, generously spread the pizza sauce all over the crust, then add a generous layer of spinach followed by your veggies. Place pizza back in the oven for 5 - 10 minutes to heat up the veggies and cook the spinach. Remove from oven and sprinkle with nutritional yeast or drizzle with cheeze sauce.

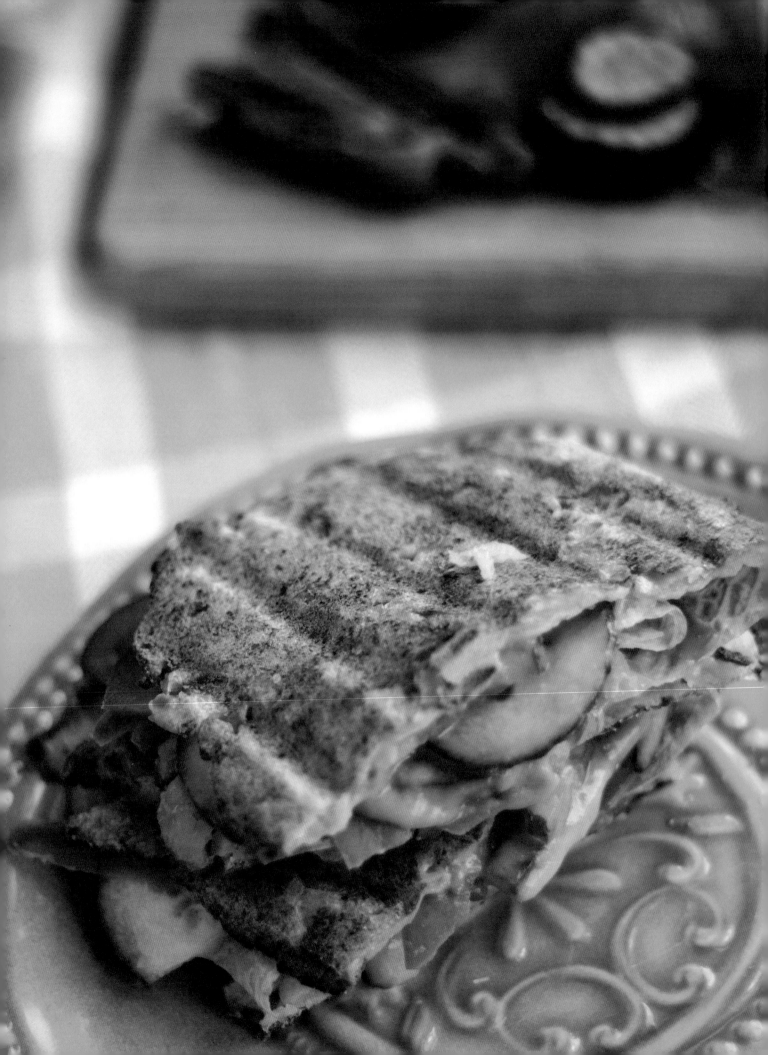

Panini Sammich

PREP TIME: 10 minutes | **COOK TIME:** 30-40 minutes | **SERVES:** 1

Ingredients

- 2-3 cups potadough
- ½ a small onion, sliced
- 4 mushrooms, sliced
- 1 bell pepper, thinly sliced
- 2 handfuls baby spinach
- 2-3 sliced sandwich pickles
- 1 cup shredded romaine or iceberg lettuce
- ¼ cup any potato cheeze sauce from this book
- 1-2 tsp mustard, optional

Good With

Fresh cut carrot, zucchini & celery sticks

Method

Line your panini maker or indoor electric grill (I use a George Foreman) with parchment paper for easy cleanup. Spread potato dough out evenly on the bottom grill plate, do not make it too thick or it will be gooey in the middle, aim for a maximum ¼-inch thick. Fill the entire bottom grill plate. Close the lid and turn on.

Not all machines have a temperature option, most default to around 400°F / 200°C. Every machine is different so it will take some experimenting on your part to get this right but generally speaking, it will take a minimum of 30 minutes for the potato dough to crisp up. Be patient, no peeking!!

If it's your first time, the sight of steam may alarm you as it looks a lot like smoke. Use your nose to tell the difference between steam and smoke. The best way to know if it's done is when there is very little to no steam coming out.

If you are in the mood for a hot sandwich, water sauté all your veggies (except for the romaine lettuce and pickles) on a non-stick pan over medium-high heat. Otherwise set veggies aside.

Remove the potato panini from the grill and cut in half. Generously spread the Potato Cheeze sauce on one half of the panini, then veggies and mustard and top with the other half of the panini. Serve and enjoy!

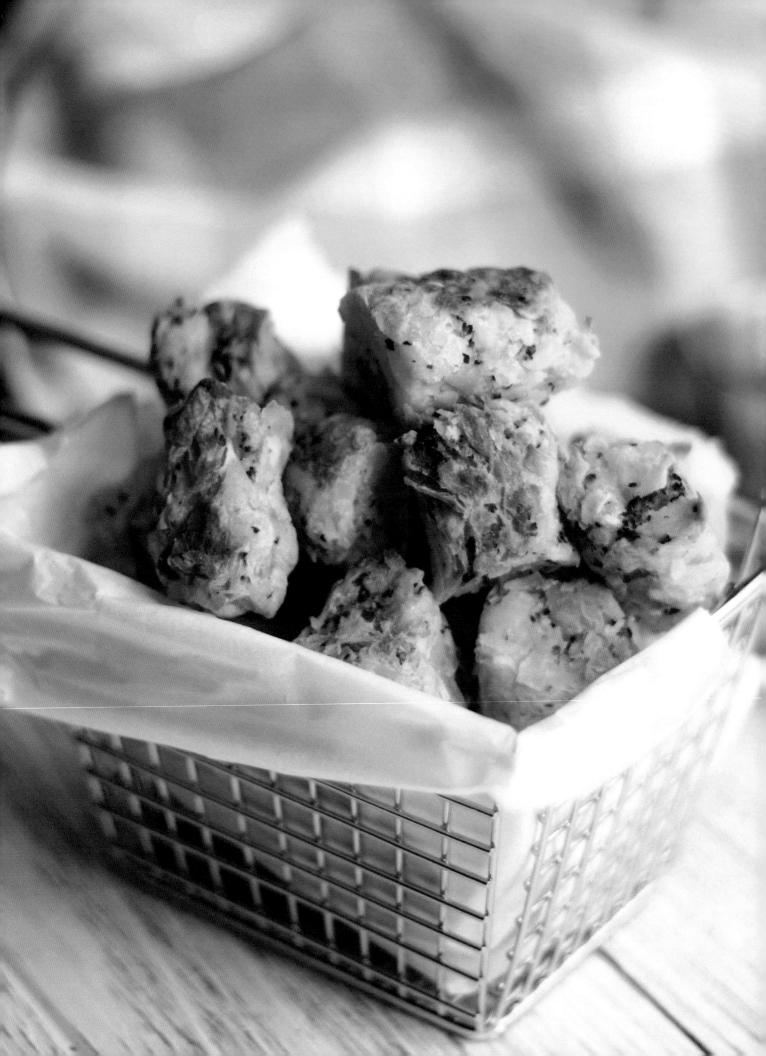

Broccoli Tots

PREP TIME: 20 minutes | **COOK TIME:** 40 minutes | **SERVES:** 1-2

Ingredients

- 4 medium leftover baked potatoes
- 1 cup broccoli, chopped
- ¼ cup nutritional yeast
- 1 tsp onion powder
- ½ tsp black pepper

Good With

No-Honey Mustard or ketchup

Method

Separate broccoli into bite sized pieces remove stems. Place broccoli florets in a small pot of water, bring to a soft boil and cook for 3 minutes. Drain, set aside and let cool.

While the broccoli is cooling off preheat oven to 450°F. Line a baking sheet with parchment paper.

In a large mixing bowl grate the potato a hand held grater. Finely chop the broccoli, then transfer to mixing bowl along with remaining ingredients. Stir until well combined.

Spoon out a heaping tablespoon of the mixture then form into a cylinder using your hands. Place onto the lined baking sheet and repeat.

Bake for 15 minutes, flip and bake for another 15-20 minutes or until golden brown.

SHORT ON TIME? Shape into patties instead of cylinders.

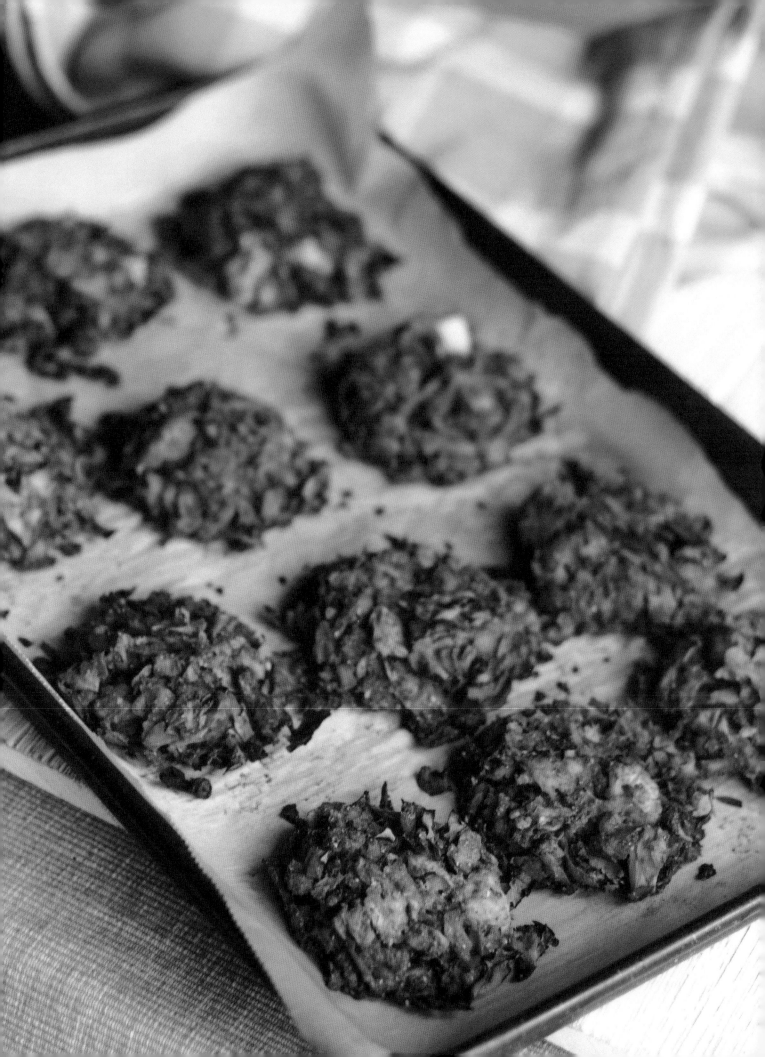

Veggie Potato Pakoras

PREP TIME: 15 minutes | **COOK TIME:** 30 minutes | **SERVES:** 1-2

Ingredients

- 4 leftover medium-sized baked potatoes
- ½ small sweet onion, diced
- 1 large carrot, shredded
- ½ cup cauliflower, diced
- 1 cup baby spinach, chopped
- 1 tsp garlic powder
- 1 tsp cumin powder
- 1 tsp yellow curry powder
- 1 tsp garam masala powder
- ½ tsp turmeric
- ¼ tsp cayenne (optional) or paprika for less heat

Good With

Smoky Sweet Mustard or No-Honey Mustard

Method

Preheat oven to 420°F. Line a baking sheet with parchment. In a small skillet, water sauté the onion, carrot, and cauliflower over medium heat for 5 minutes – add water as necessary to prevent sticking. Stir in the dry spices and spinach then cover, continue cooking for another 5 minutes.

While the veggies are cooking: shred the leftover baked potatoes in a large mixing bowl.

Add the sautéed veggies to the shredded potatoes and stir well to combine.

Using your hands, or a small measuring cup and press into patties. It's important that the mixture forms well and sticks together. Place pakoras on the parchment lined baking sheet.

Bake for 20 to 30 minutes until crispy on the outside.

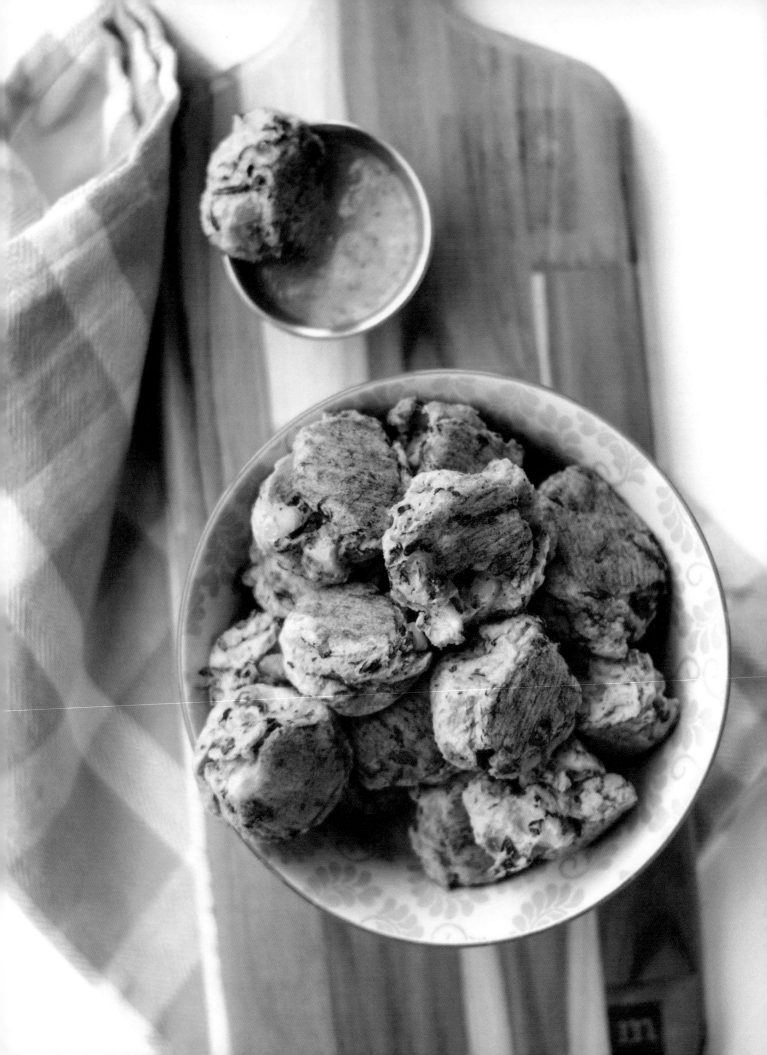

Colcannon Puffs

PREP TIME: 10 minutes | **COOK TIME:** 45 minutes | **SERVES:** 1-2

Ingredients

- 4 medium potatoes
- 2 cups raw baby spinach or steamed kale, finely chopped
- 2 tbsp nutritional yeast
- 1 tsp garlic powder
- 1 tsp onion powder
- ½ tsp Italian seasoning
- ¼ tsp black pepper

Good With

No-Honey Mustard or Ketchup

Method

Wash, peel and cut your potatoes into quarters, or smaller. Place in a large pot and cover with water. Bring to a boil and cook until potatoes are tender.

While the potatoes are cooking, prepare the spinach – chop finely. If you're using kale instead, you'll need to remove the stems, and lightly steam or boil (you can place it in the potato water for a few minutes and remove with a slotted spoon.) Drain the water from the potatoes.

Preheat oven to 420°F. Line a baking sheet with parchment paper.

Mash the potatoes using a hand masher, don't worry if it's not perfectly smooth. Stir in remaining nutritional yeast and spices. We are purposely not using any liquid for this mash. Scoop out a heaping tablespoon and form into ball with hands and place onto a parchment lined baking sheet, repeat.

Bake for 15 minutes, flip and bake for another 15 minutes or until desired crispness.

DID YOU KNOW? Colcannon is a traditional Irish dish of mashed potatoes with kale or cabbage. It can contain other ingredients such as scallions, leeks, onions and chives.

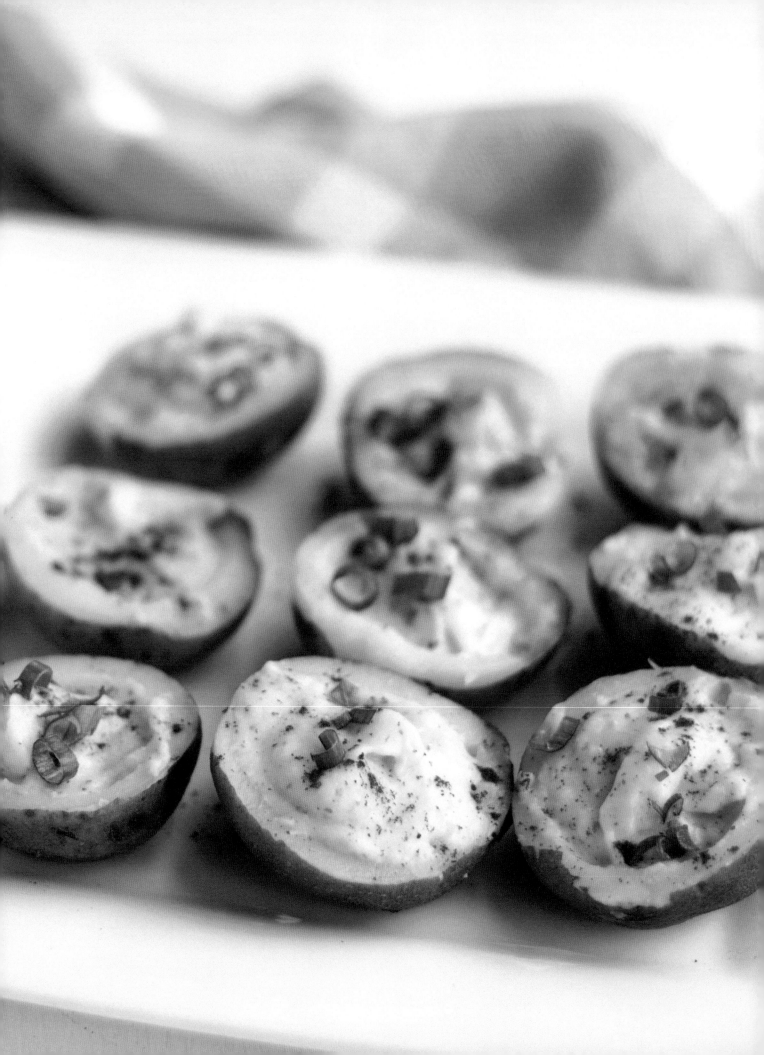

Little Devils

PREP TIME: 30 minutes | **COOK TIME:** 20 minutes | **SERVES:** 1-2

Ingredients

- 6 small blemish-free red potatoes
- 1 tbsp stone ground or dijon mustard
- 1 tsp yellow mustard
- ½ tsp garlic powder
- 1 tsp onion powder
- 1 bunch chives or 1 green onion, finely chopped
- paprika & black pepper and low sodium salt, to taste

Good With

Large leafy green salad or Hearty Veggie Soup

Method

Wash and remove any dirt from potatoes. Boil potatoes until fork-tender. Drain and let cool completely. To speed up this process cool in the fridge or freezer – just don't forget about them if you put them in the freezer.

Once the potatoes are cool, slice in half lengthwise. Using a spoon, score a border on the flesh approximately ¼ of an inch in from the edge of the potato, then scoop out most of the potato flesh leaving behind ¼ of an inch of flesh attached to the skin. Set skins aside.

Place the scooped out potato guts into a medium bowl and mash with mustards, garlic powder and onion powder. Mash with a fork until smooth and fluffy. Do not use an immersion blender for as it will make the potato mixture stiff and gluey.

Spoon the potato mixture back into the skins. Garnish with chives, paprika and black pepper..

GET FANCY! Make this look pretty by squeezing the potato mixture through one of those fancy pastry or piping bags for cake decorating.

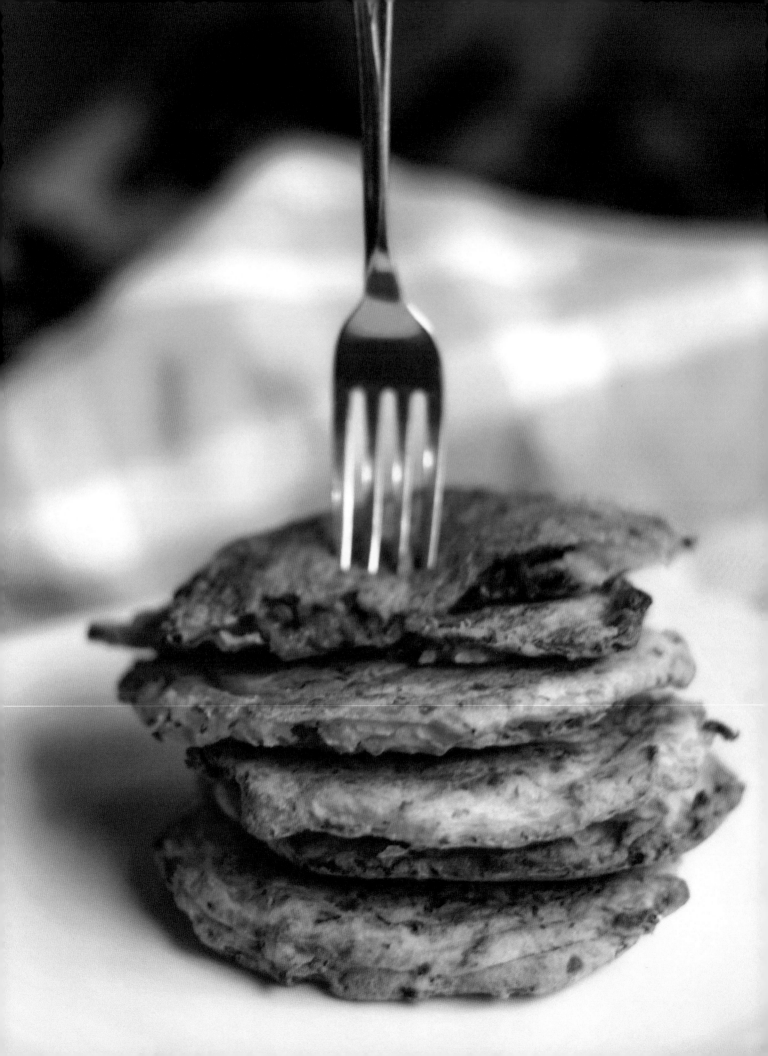

Stuffed Potato Cakes

PREP TIME: 10 minutes | **COOK TIME:** 50-60 minutes | **SERVES:** 1-2

Ingredients

- 4 cups mashed potatoes, stiff mixture, or potadough
- 1½ tbsp potato flour
- 3 tbsp nutritional yeast
- 1 tsp garlic powder
- 1 tsp Italian seasoning
- 2 tsp dried parsley pepper and salt (optional) to taste

FILLING

- 12 white or brown mushrooms, finely chopped
- ½ white onion, finely chopped
- ¼ cup red bell pepper, finely chopped
- 3 cups fresh spinach, finely chopped
- 1 tbsp dried parsley
- ½ tbsp Italian seasoning

Method

Preheat oven to 425°F. Line a baking sheet with parchment paper.

In a skillet, water sauté the onion, mushrooms and bell pepper over medium heat until tender – add water as necessary to prevent sticking. Stir in the spinach, parsley and Italian seasoning and continue sautéing for 3 minutes. Remove from heat, drain off any excess liquid, set aside.

In a large bowl, using your hands, combine mashed potatoes, potato flour, nutritional yeast, garlic powder and parsley. Then separate your "dough" in 12 equal sized balls. Form six balls into thin patties and place on the parchment lined baking sheet. Put 1-2 tablespoons of the filling into the middle of each patty. From the remaining dough, form six more thin patties and place on top of the filling, pinch sides to seal it.

Sprinkle with pepper and optional salt. Bake for 30 min, carefully, turn over, bake another 20-30 min until outside is good and crunchy.

CHEF'S NOTE: My fillings are just a suggestion but they pair very well with potatoes. As always, feel free to make it your own and add your own favorites. That's what makes cooking fun, isn't it?

RECIPE PROVIDED BY COOKING WITH MARY
You can find this and many more delicious plant based recipes here: cookingwithmaryplantbased.weebly.com

Everything Potato Bagels

PREP TIME: Overnight | **COOK TIME: 20 minutes** | **SERVES: 1-3**

Ingredients

- 2-3 cups potadough
- ¼ cup nutritional yeast (optional)
- ¼ tsp salt (optional)
- 1 donut or muffin pan

"EVERYTHING" SEASONING

- 1-2 tsp sea salt flakes or other coarse salt
- 4 tbsp minced dried garlic
- 4 tbsp dried onion flakes
- ¼-½ tsp ground caraway (optional)

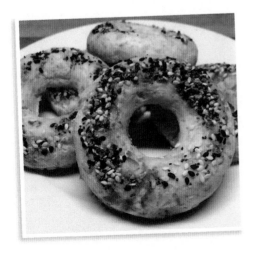

Method

Seasoning: Mix together and store any leftovers in an airtight container.

Dough: you can use leftover mashed potatoes, potadough or the innards from freshly baked potatoes. Optionally, mash in some nutritional yeast for a cheesy flavor.

Sprinkle the Everything seasoning in the bottom of a donut pan, then press the potatoes into the pan on top of the seasoning, packing in well with a spoon or spatula. Chill for 8-12 hours.

Preheat oven to 400°F. Flip chilled potatoes onto a parchment lined baking sheet. Bake for 15-20 minutes, they should be golden and crisp on the outside. Best when served immediately. You can also re-crisp them for a few minutes if they cool and get soft.

NO DONUT PAN? If you don't have a donut pan, you can just use a muffin pan and hollow out the middle a bit. They will still taste just as good.

NOTE: Keep in mind that these are basically potato nuggets and not chewy bread like an actual bagel. They aren't going to function the same way, but are an awesome way to get a potato powered, flour free, everything bagel flavor fix! ~ Pebbles

RECIPE & PHOTO PROVIDED BY PEBBLES EATS PLANTS
You can find this and many more delicious plant based recipes here: pebbleseatsplants.com

istockphoto.com

Potato Taco Shells

PREP TIME: 10 | **COOK TIME:** 10 minutes | **SERVES:** 1-2

Ingredients

FILLING INGREDIENTS:

7   Large button mushrooms diced

¼   medium onion diced

4   small precooked potatoes diced for filling

1   tsp or more taco seasonings of your choice to taste

SHELL INGREDIENTS:

12   tiny potatoes or 4 medium potatoes for shell

TOPPINGS:

Nacho Cheeze Sauce

Method

In a large sauté pan over medium heat cook mushrooms, onions and potatoes until cooked through. Add any taco seasoning of your choice. Set aside.

Slice potatoes thin on a mandolin. Arrange slices on a microwave chip maker, overlapping to form the size taco shell you want. I cooked mine in the microwave for 4 minutes. You want it done enough to hold together but not so crisp it can't be formed. Remove from microwave and fold over to form taco shell. I used a paper towel holder as a form. Use whatever can be safely put into the microwave. Now return shell to microwave and cook until crisp. I cooked mine another 2 minutes but of course microwaves vary. Repeat to make 3 more shells, depending on the size you want you may get more or less.

Now just add your filling, toppings and cheeze sauce.

NOTE: I've heard from many fellow spuddies that the Chiptastic chip maker for the microwave works really well

RECIPE & PHOTO PROVIDED BY KARI EATS PLANTS
You can find this and many more delicious plant based recipes here: karieatsplants.wordpress.com

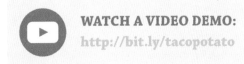

WATCH A VIDEO DEMO:
http://bit.ly/tacopotato

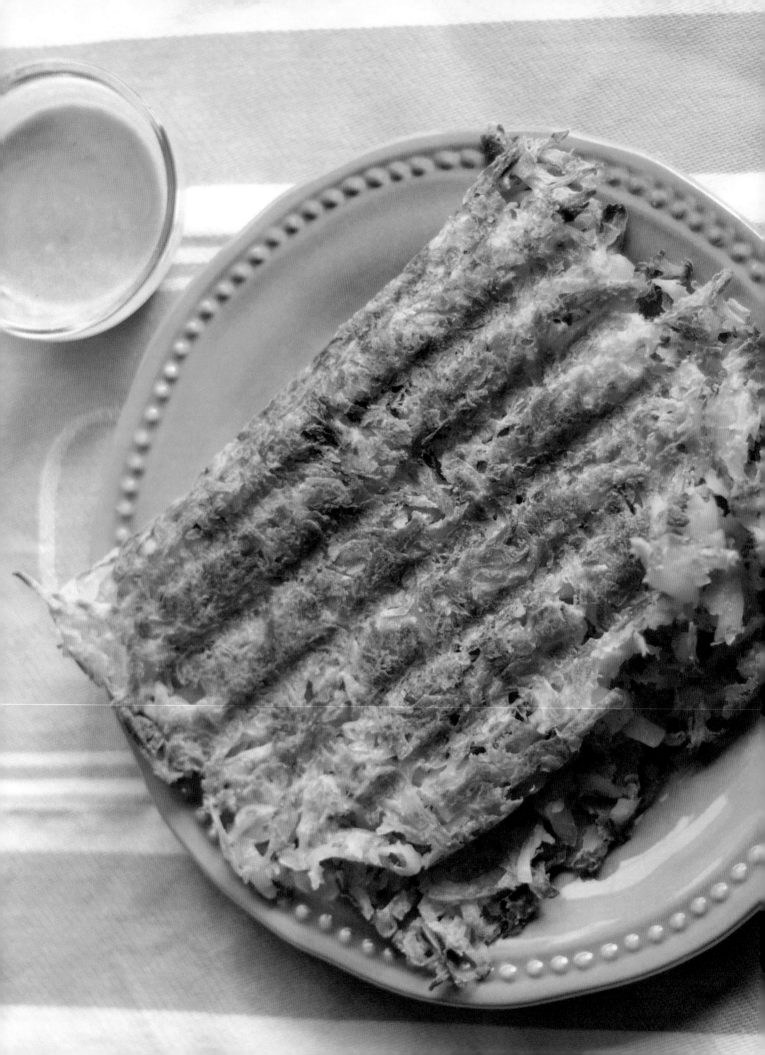

Crispy Hash Browns

PREP TIME: 5 minutes | **COOK TIME:** 30 minutes | **SERVES:** 1-2

Ingredients

- 4 medium, or 2 large leftover cold baked potatoes
- 1 handful of chopped spinach or broccoli slaw
- 1 tsp of your favorite spice combo

Good With

Lettuce wraps & No-Honey Mustard

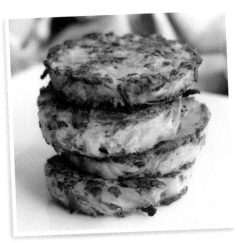

Method

Preheat oven to 420°F. Line a baking sheet with parchment paper.

Shred the potatoes, using a hand held grater, into a large mixing bowl. Toss together shredded potatoes, spices and chopped spinach or broccoli slaw. Transfer to the parchment lined baking sheet, spreading out evenly.

Bake for 30 minutes or until desired crispiness. Cooking time varies oven to oven, so keep a close eye after 20 minutes.

ELECTRIC GRILL OPTION: These come out just as good on an electric grill such as a George Foreman grill or panini maker. Because of the variations in brands and grill types, I can only give you a general idea on cooking time. On my grill it takes 30 minutes for the hash browns to crisp up and not stick. If there's a lot of steam coming out of your grill it's not ready.

MAKE THEM INTO FUN SHAPES!
I pressed these into a measuring cup before placing on baking sheet.

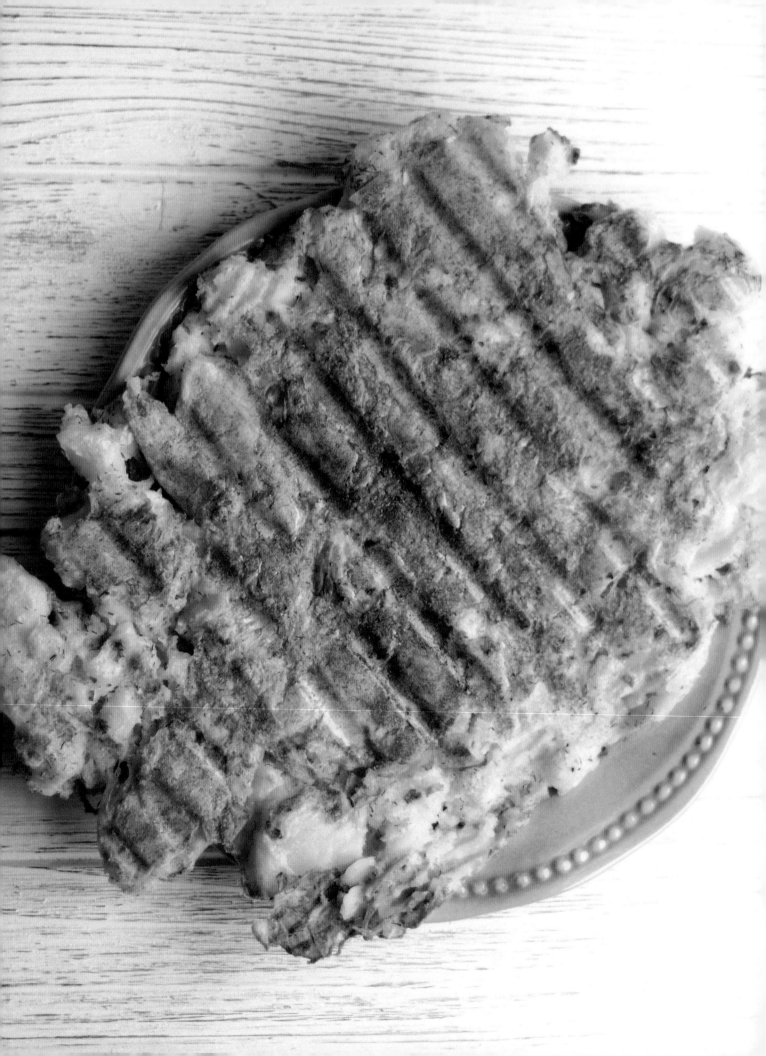

Grilled Potato Pancakes

PREP TIME: 5 minutes | **COOK TIME:** 30 minutes | **SERVES:** 1

Ingredients

- 2-3   cups potadough
- 1   tsp spices of your choice (optional)

Good With

Side salad & any potato cheeze sauce from this book

WATCH A VIDEO DEMO:

http://bit.ly/
potatocakesrecipe

Method

Using your hands or a wooden spoon mix spices into your pre-made potato dough. Spread the potato dough onto a George Foreman grill or similar, press down with your fingers until no more than ¼" thick. Close the lid and turn on.

Close the lid and cook for approximately 30 minutes, or until there's very little steam coming out. If your machine has a temperature option, set it to around 400°F/200°C. No peeking! Avoid opening the lid part-way through.

If it's your first time, the sight of steam may alarm you as it looks a lot like smoke. Use your nose to tell the difference between steam and smoke.

Sometimes, depending on how wet your dough mixture is, it can take up to 40 minutes for mine to crisp up. The best way to know if it's done is when the steam is gone.

TIP: If you're afraid of messing it up and having a stuck-on mess, or if you're like me and like easy clean up, you can line your grill with parchment paper. It crisps up just the same!

IN A HURRY AND NO MASHED POTATOES? Bake a few potatoes in the microwave, roughly mash with a fork without any liquid then cook on grill machine for approximately 15 minutes.

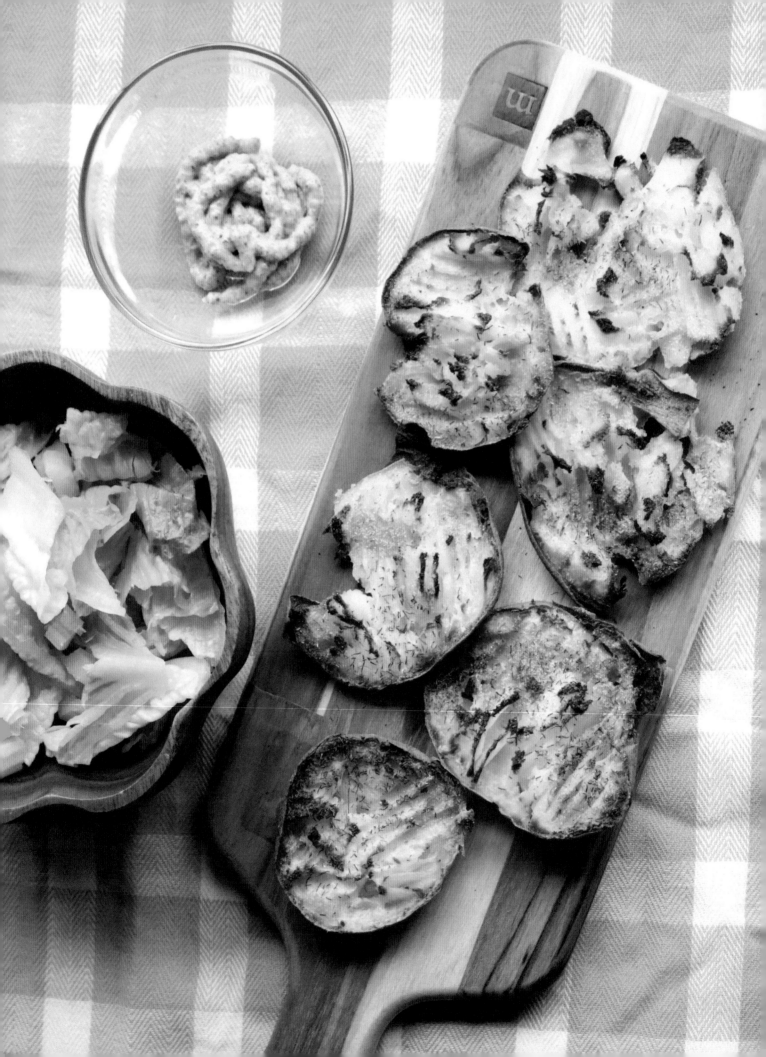

Crispy Smashed Potatoes

PREP TIME: 10 minutes | **COOK TIME:** 20 minutes | **SERVES:** 1

Ingredients

- 4 medium leftover baked potatoes
- ½ tsp smoked paprika
- ½ tsp garlic powder
  or
- 1 tsp of your favorite spice combo

Good With

Ketchup, mustard, gravy or potato cheeze sauce

Method

Preheat oven to 420°F. Line a baking sheet with parchment paper.

Cut the leftover baked potatoes in half lengthwise, and arrange, flesh-side up on the parchment-lined baking sheet. Smash each potato with a fork.

Sprinkle potatoes with smoked paprika and garlic powder. Bake for 20 minutes or until crisp.

NO BAKED POTATOES ON HAND? Bake a them in the microwave. Same rules apply, wash and poke holes before cooking. Microwave times vary, cook in 3-minute increments until all potatoes are soft.

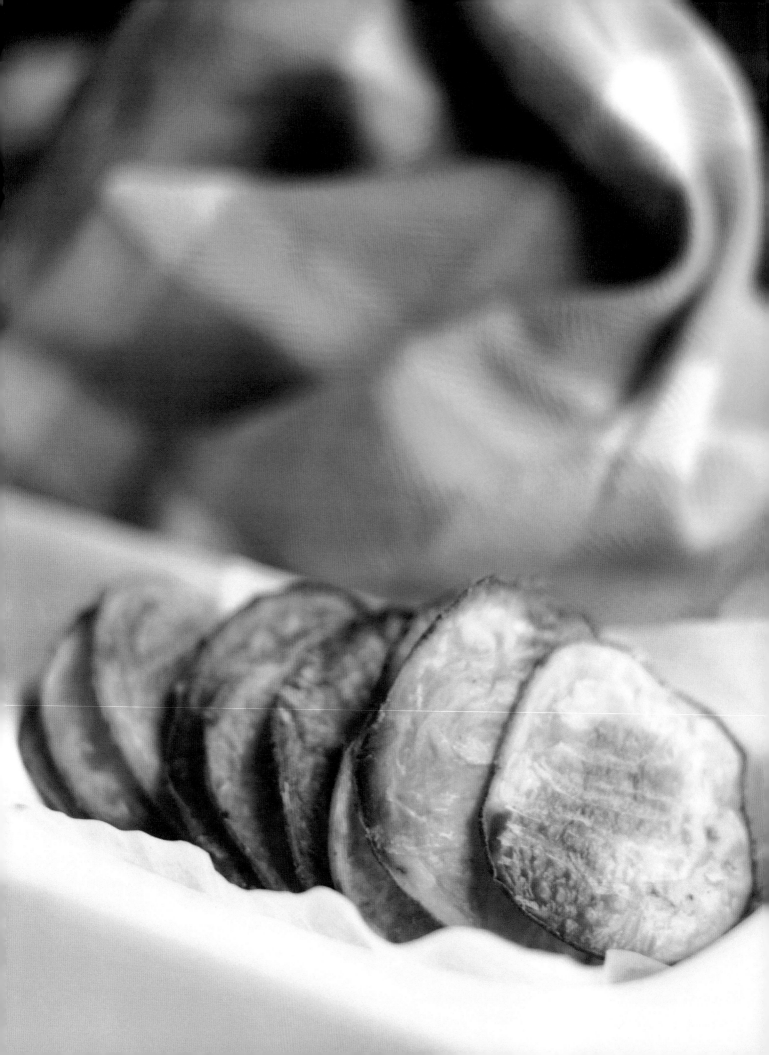

Crispy Potato Chips

PREP TIME: 10 minutes | **COOK TIME:** 15-30 minutes | **SERVES:** 1

Ingredients

- 2 medium russet potatoes
- 1 tsp of your favorite spices

Good With

Fresh cut veggies and Potato Ranch Dip

Method

Preheat oven to 400°F. Line two baking sheets with parchment paper.

Wash potatoes, remove blemishes and pat dry. Carefully and evenly cut into thin slices – a good quality mandolin will speed up this process and create evenly cut slices.

In a large bowl, toss in spices and potatoes together using your hands.

Spread the potato slices on the parchment lined baking sheets so they are not overlapping.

Bake for 15 minutes, flip, bake for another 10-15 minutes or until crisp. Keep a close eye on them as they can burn very easily.

NOTE: I've heard from many fellow spuddies that the Chiptastic chip maker for the microwave works really well, and quickly!

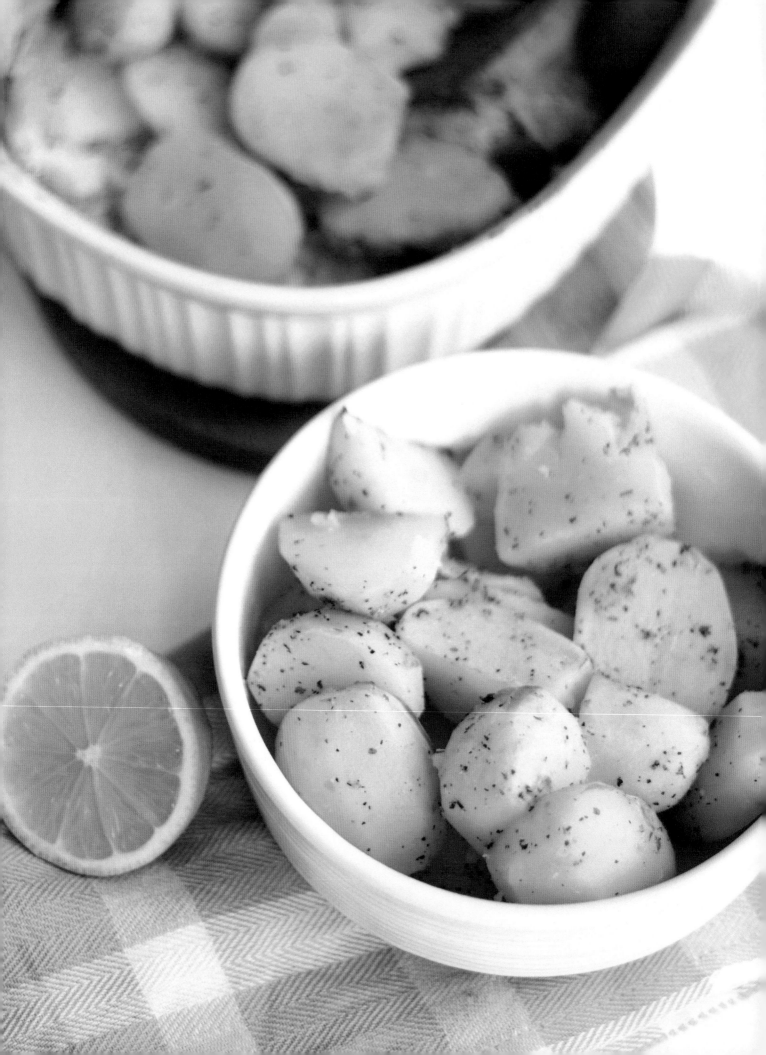

Lemony Greek Potatoes

PREP TIME: 5 minutes | **COOK TIME:** 60-65 minutes | **SERVES:** 2

Ingredients

- 4 large Yukon gold potatoes
- ¾ cup water
- 2 lemons
- ½ tsp garlic powder
- ½ tsp onion powder
- ½ tsp dried oregano
- ¼ tsp black pepper

Good With

A large leafy green salad with House Dressing 2.0

Method

Preheat oven to 350°F. Peel and rinse potatoes.

Cut potatoes into quarters and place in a large bowl along with the juice of 1 lemons and spices in a large bowl, combine well with hands.

Pour potato mixture into to a glass baking dish or casserole dish. Next, pour the water into the corner of the baking dish – NOT over the potatoes or you will end up rinsing the lemon and spices off the potatoes.

Cover dish with aluminum foil or oven-safe lid. Bake for 45 minutes or until soft.

Remove foil/lid, turn the heat up to 425°F and continue baking for another 15-20 minutes or until edges start to brown.

Cut the remaining lemon into wedges to squeeze over potatoes as desired.

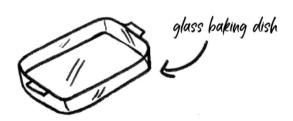

glass baking dish

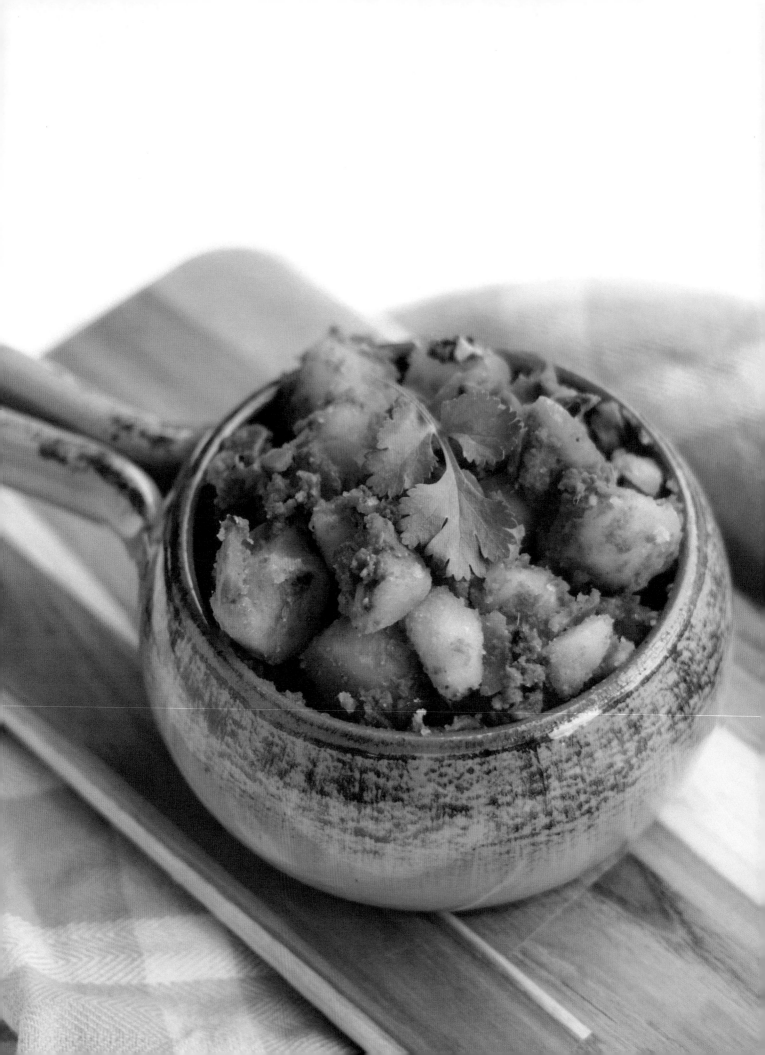

Bombay Pan Potatoes

PREP TIME: 15 minutes | **COOK TIME: 40 minutes** | **SERVES: 1-2**

Ingredients

- 3 large potatoes, cubed
- 1 14.5-oz can no-salt-added diced tomatoes
- 1" fresh ginger, peeled
- 2 garlic cloves, peeled
- 1 tsp cumin seeds
- 1 large yellow onion, chopped
- 1 tsp turmeric
- 2 tsp ground coriander
- 1 tsp ground cumin
- 1 tsp garam masala
- 1 tsp paprika or if you like spicy: a pinch of cayenne pepper
- 1 tbsp fresh coriander (cilantro) leaves

Method

Wash, peel and chop potatoes into ½-inch cubes. Place in a large pot, cover with water and boil until tender (20-30 minutes). Drain and set aside.

While the potatoes are cooking: place the ginger, garlic and half a can of the diced tomatoes in a blender. Blend until smooth. Set aside.

Add the cumin seeds to a large frying pan and toast over medium-high heat for a minute or two. Stir often to prevent burning. Add the onion and a thin layer of water, sauté until onion is soft. Then add the tomato, ginger, garlic mixture along with turmeric, ground coriander, ground cumin, garam masala and paprika. Continue sautéing for two more minutes.

Add the remaining half can of diced tomatoes, stir well and cook until tomatoes soften (approximately two minutes). Carefully add in the potatoes and cook for another five minutes. Stir in the chopped coriander and serve.

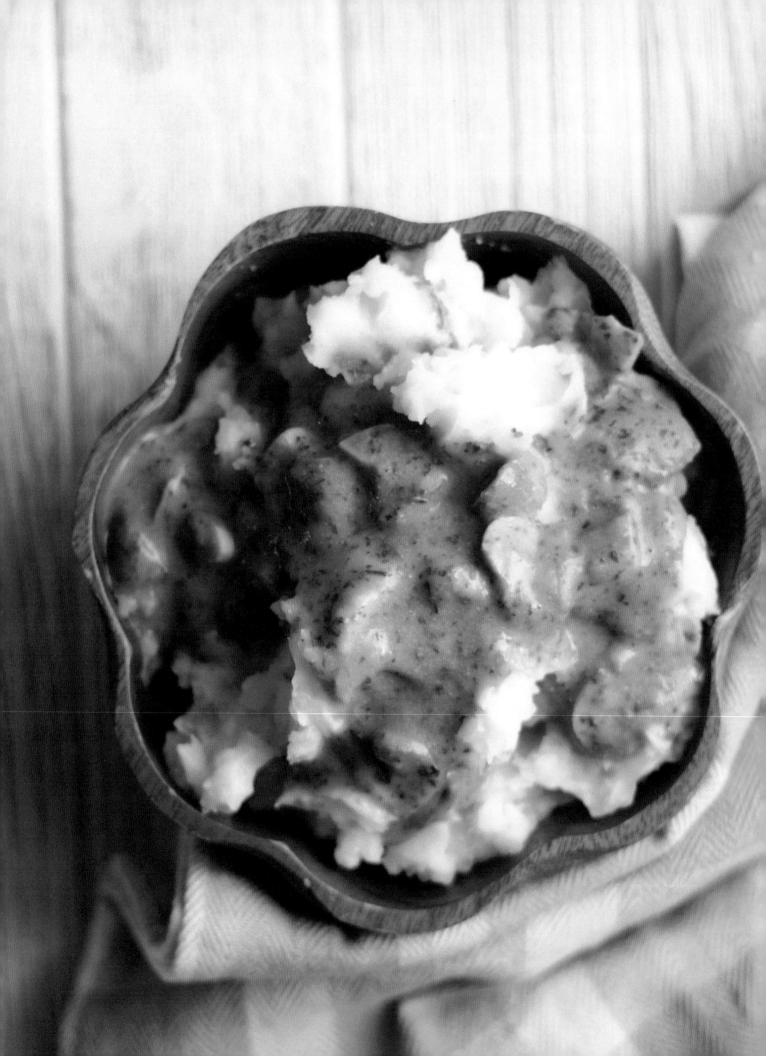

Creamy Mashed Potatoes

PREP TIME: 5 minutes | **COOK TIME:** 30 minutes | **SERVES:** 2

Ingredients

- 4 medium golden potatoes
- ¼ cup no-salt-added vegetable broth or unsweetened non-dairy milk
- ½ tsp garlic powder
- ½ tsp onion powder
- ¼ cup chives or green onion, chopped, for garnish

Good With

Steamed veggies and golden gravy

Method

Wash, peel (optional) and cut your potatoes into quarters. Place in a stock pot and cover with water. Cook over high heat until potatoes are fork tender. Watch that the water does not boil over; reduce heat slightly if necessary.

Carefully drain water. Add spices to potatoes and mash while gradually adding the broth or potato water as necessary, until you achieve the consistency you prefer.

TIP: I don't recommend an immersion blender (sharp blades) for mashing because it's very easy to over mix and become very gluey. Instead, use a hand masher or electric mixer (for whisking and beating).

GET CREATIVE WITH SPICES! Don't be afraid to try out different spice combinations. Just be sure to not accidentally dump half a cup of chili powder into your mashed potatoes like I did!

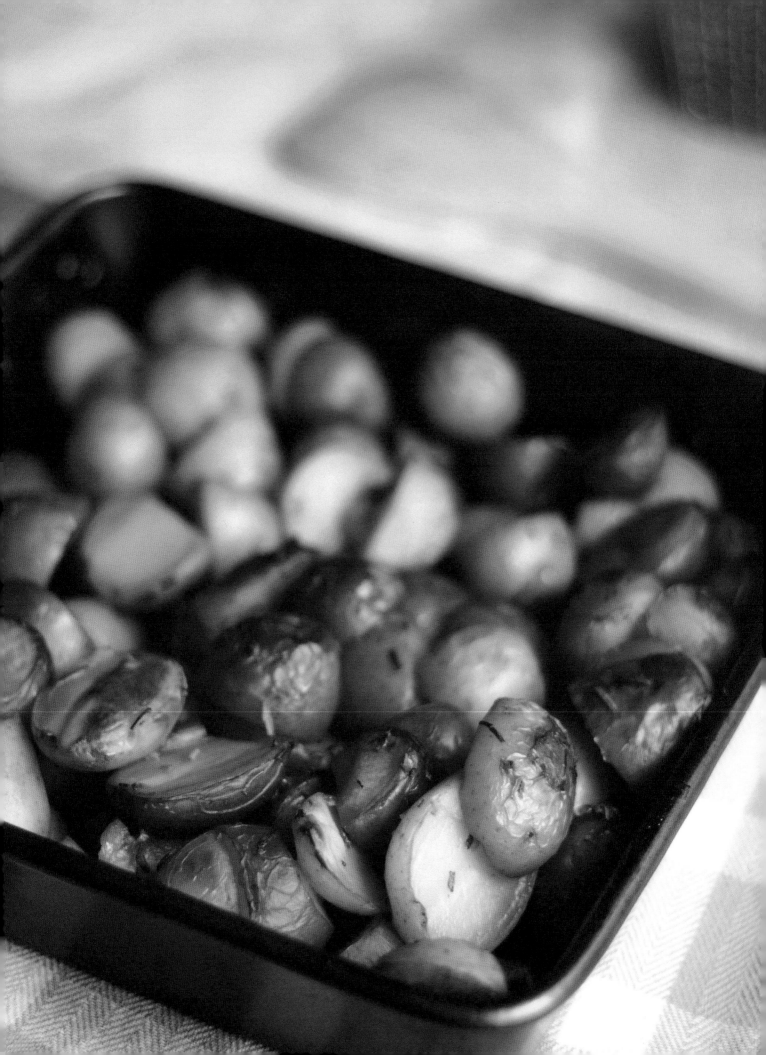

Roasted Rosemary Garlic Potatoes

PREP TIME: 10 minutes | **COOK TIME: 55-60 minutes** | **SERVES: 1-3**

Ingredients

- 2 lbs baby potatoes, halved
- 1 cup no-salt added vegetable broth, divided
- 2 garlic cloves, minced
- ½ tbsp potato starch
- ¼ tsp dried rosemary

Good With

Roasted veggies of your choice

Method

Preheat oven to 400°F. Wash and gently scrub any dirt off the potatoes. Cut potatoes in half, or if some are larger than others quarters if necessary – so that they are all approximately the same size.

In a small saucepan whisk ½ cup of the vegetable broth with the potato starch to combine well. Add in the garlic and dried herbs and bring to a boil to thicken. Remove from heat.

In a large mixing bowl coat potatoes in the thickened broth mixture. Line a casserole dish or roasting pan with the remaining ½ cup of vegetable broth – enough broth to thinly coat the bottom of the dish, then add potatoes. Bake, covered, for 40 minutes. Remove lid, stir potatoes and increase oven temperature to 450°F. Continue cooking uncovered for 15-20 minutes or until golden brown.

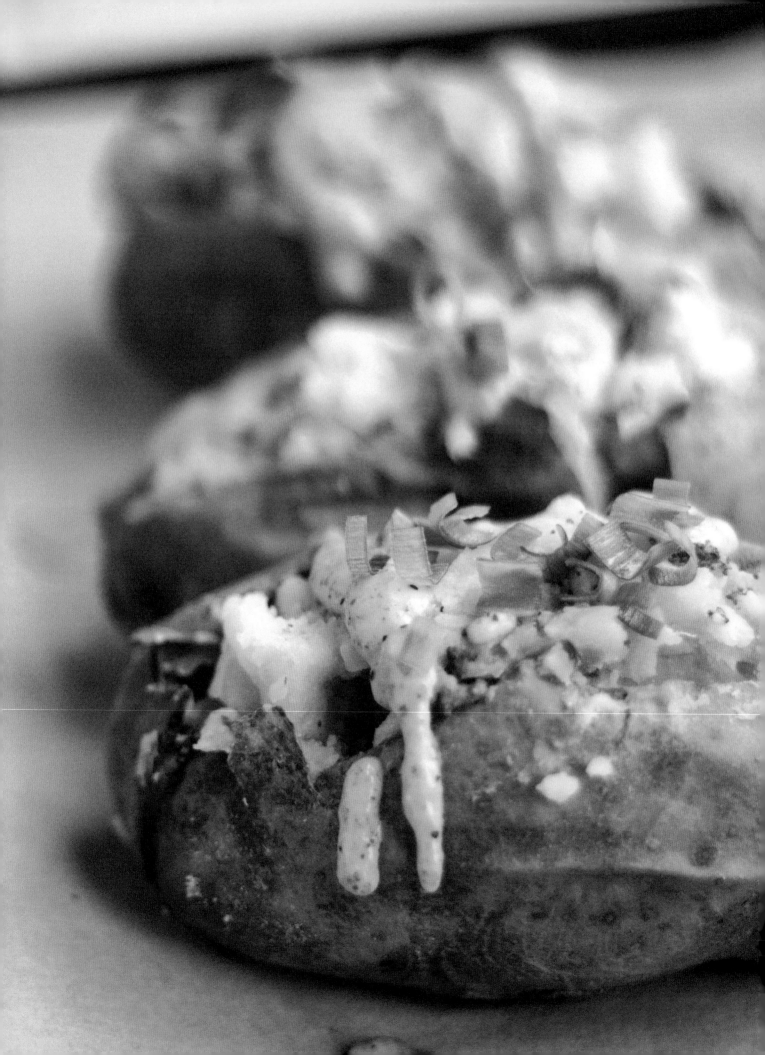

Twice Baked Potatoes

PREP TIME: 10 minutes | **COOK TIME:** 55-70 minutes | **SERVES:** 1-2

Ingredients

- 2 large russet potatoes
- ½ tsp onion powder
- ½ tsp garlic powder
- 1 cup broccoli or cauliflower, chopped
- 2-3 tbsp unsweetened non-dairy milk or no-salt added vegetable broth
- 1 green onion, chopped
- ½ tsp smoked paprika

Good With

Any potato cheese sauce from this book

Method

Preheat oven to 425°F. Wash potatoes and pierce each potato several times with a fork. Place on a parchment lined baking sheet. Bake for 45-60 minutes or until soft.

Meanwhile, steam, boil or microwave the broccoli until soft. Mash with a fork to break it up into small pieces, set aside.

Remove baked potatoes from oven and carefully cut in half, lengthwise, with a sharp knife. Then with a potholder or oven mit, cradle one of the potato halves in palm of your hand over a large bowl and scrape out the potato guts using a spoon. Be careful not to scrape through the skin. Place emptied potatoes back on the parchment lined baking sheet. Repeat until you have scraped out all the potato guts.

Add onion powder, garlic powder and non-dairy milk to the potato guts. Mash until smooth using a potato masher or fork, then stir in the cooked broccoli. Scoop mashed potatoes back into the potato shells. Return to oven and bake for 10 minutes.

Sprinkle with green onions, smoked paprika and if desired drizzle with potato cheese sauce.

FANCY VERSION: Instead of cutting potatoes in half, cut a wedge from the potato, then remove the potato guts.

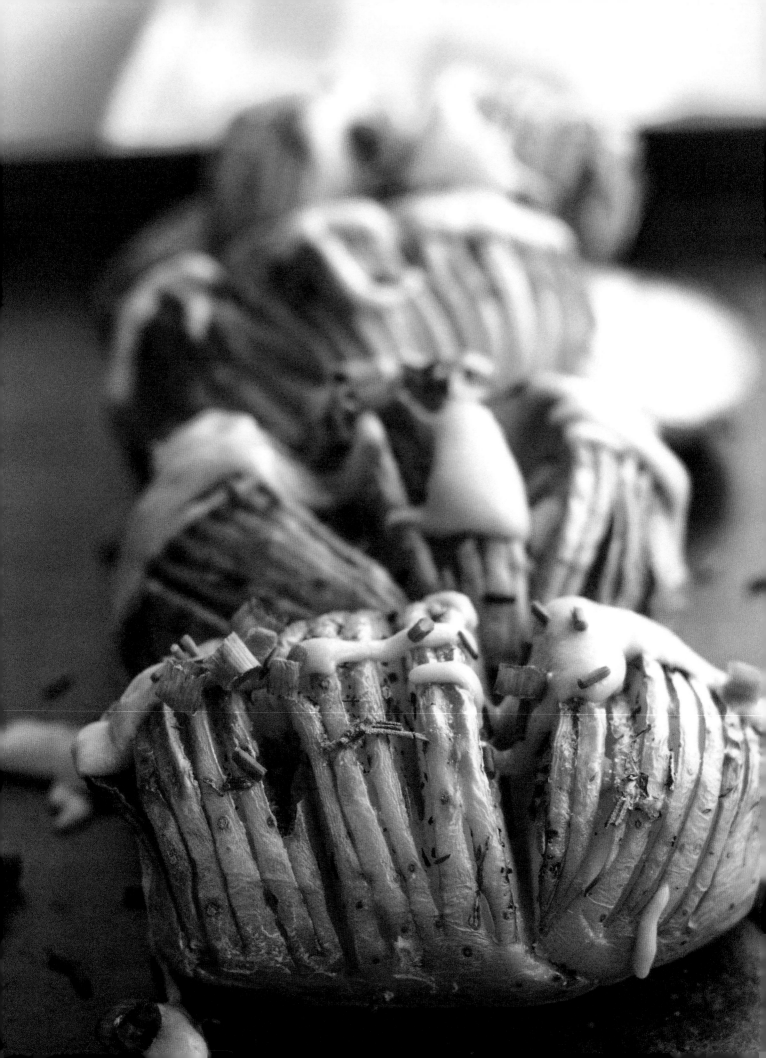

Hasselback Potatoes

PREP TIME: 15 minutes | **COOK TIME:** 60 minutes | **SERVES:** 1-2

Ingredients

- 4 medium gold or russet potatoes
- ⅔ cup no-salt-added vegetable broth
- 2 garlic cloves, minced
- ½ tbsp potato starch
- ¼ tsp dried rosemary
- ¼ tsp dried thyme

Good With

Steamed vegetables with Unicorn Dust

Method

Preheat oven to 420°F. Wash and dry the potatoes well; do not peel.

Cut narrow slices into the potatoes, approximately 3/4 of the way down – don't cut all the way through. Spread apart the slices a little as you go. If you need a more stable surface, slice a small amount off the bottoms so they sit flat. Place sliced potatoes on a parchment-lined baking sheet.

In a small saucepan, whisk together the potato starch and veggie broth. Stir in the garlic and dried herbs. Bring to a boil, stirring until it thickens. Set aside.

Brush the potatoes with the thickened veggie broth mixture. Bake for 30 minutes. Brush the potatoes with the remaining veggie broth mixture. Bake for an additional 30 minutes or until soft on the inside and golden brown on the outside.

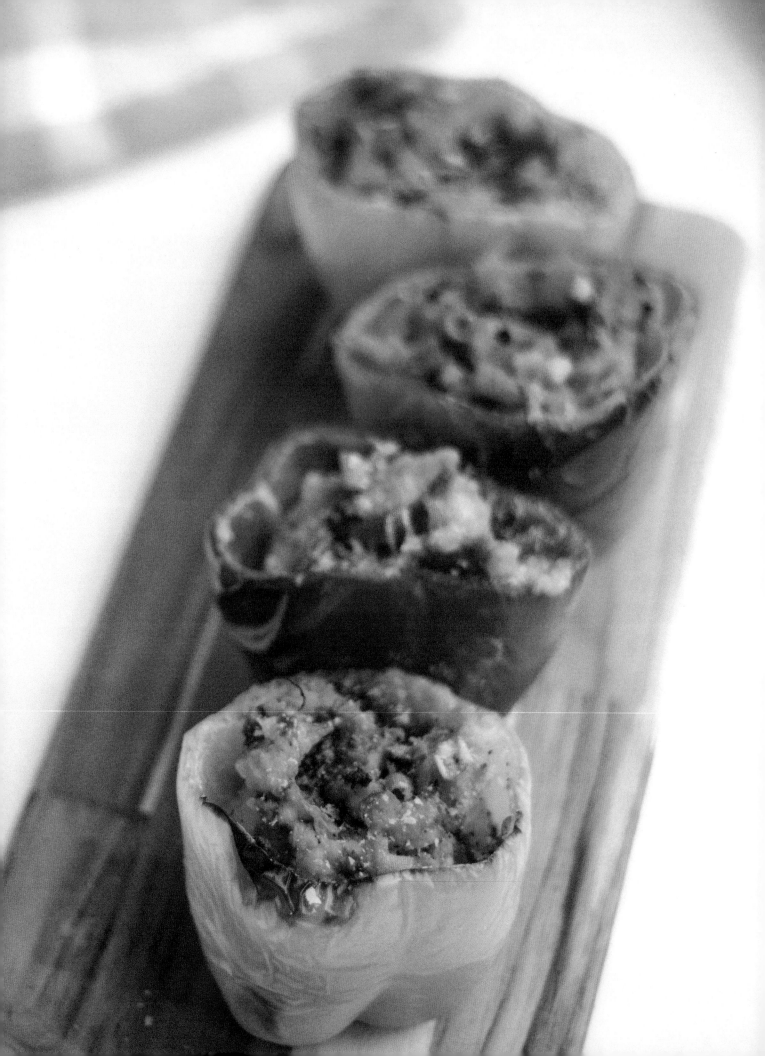

Potato Stuffed Peppers

PREP TIME: 10 minutes | **COOK TIME:** 35-45 minutes | **SERVES:** 1-3

Ingredients

- 2 red bell peppers
- 1 medium sweet potato
- 2 medium yellow potatoes
- 2 tbsp nutritional yeast
- 1 tsp garlic powder
- 1 tsp onion powder

Good With

Large leafy green salad with House Dressing 2.0

Method

Preheat oven to 350°F. Cut the tops off or halve the bell peppers. Remove seeds and membranes, rinse peppers. Place empty peppers on a parchment lined baking sheet and bake for 15 minutes. Remove from oven and set aside to let cool.

While the peppers are baking: wash, peel and cut potatoes. Boil or pressure cook potatoes until soft. Drain. Mash with nutritional yeast, garlic powder and onion powder, and if needed, add a splash of vegetable broth.

Stuff peppers with mashed potato mixture and place back on the parchment lined baking sheet. Bake for 20-30 minutes until peppers are soft and beginning to brown.

AIR FRYER VERSION: Place the stuffed peppers in an air fryer for 20-30 minutes, until peppers are soft and beginning to brown.

TIP: to save time, use leftover potatoes for the stuffing.

Boiled Taters & Dill

PREP TIME: 10 minutes | **COOK TIME:** 20 minutes | **SERVES:** 1-2

Ingredients

4	medium red or yellow potatoes
½	lemon
½	tsp onion powder
½	tsp garlic powder
1	tsp dried or fresh dill
	black pepper to taste, optional

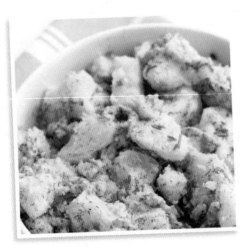

Method

Wash, peel (optional) and chop potatoes into quarters or smaller chunks, depending on your preference. Boil potatoes until tender, drain.

Squeeze lemon juice over potatoes, sprinkle with spices, dill and black pepper. Serve and enjoy!

NOT INTO DILL? Try it with chopped fresh chives or green onions.

TO PEEL OR NOT TO PEEL? I personally find boiled potatoes with skins unap*peeling*, it's a texture thing. We all know that the skins are good for us, but if there's ever a time you're just not in the mood for them go ahead and peel!

Potato Salad

PREP TIME: 10 minutes | **COOK TIME:** 20 minutes | **SERVES:** 3-4

Ingredients

5	medium red potatoes
1	stalk celery
1	green onion
1	garlic clove, skinned
2	tbsp dijon mustard
1	tbsp apple cider vinegar
½	tbsp dried dill
½	tbsp pure maple syrup
1	tsp onion powder
¼	cup potato water
¼	tsp reduced sodium salt
	paprika & black pepper to taste

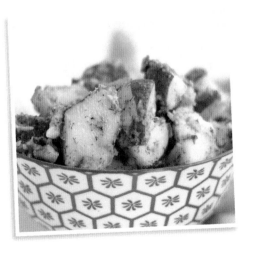

Method

Wash potatoes and remove blemishes. Cut into 1" cubes and add to a large stock pot. Cover with water and bring to a boil. Cook until just *barely* fork tender. Careful not to overcook, we don't want a mushy potato for potato salad.

While the potatoes are cooking, dice the celery and green onion.

With a mug or glass measuring cup, scoop out approximately half a cup of the potato cooking water, set aside. Drain potatoes and set aside. Scoop out ¾ cup of the potatoes and place in a blender. Place the remaining potatoes in large mixing bowl.

In a blender with the ¾ cup of potatoes add mustard, apple cider vinegar, ¼ cup potato water, maple syrup, garlic clove and onion powder. Blend until smooth. Add more potato water if necessary. It should be the consistency of a creamy salad dressing.

Mix together potatoes with dressing, diced onion, celery and dill. Top with black pepper and paprika. Let cool in fridge for at least one hour.

NOTE: This recipe was adapted from High Carb Hannah's Creamy Potato Salad from PlantMealPlanner.com

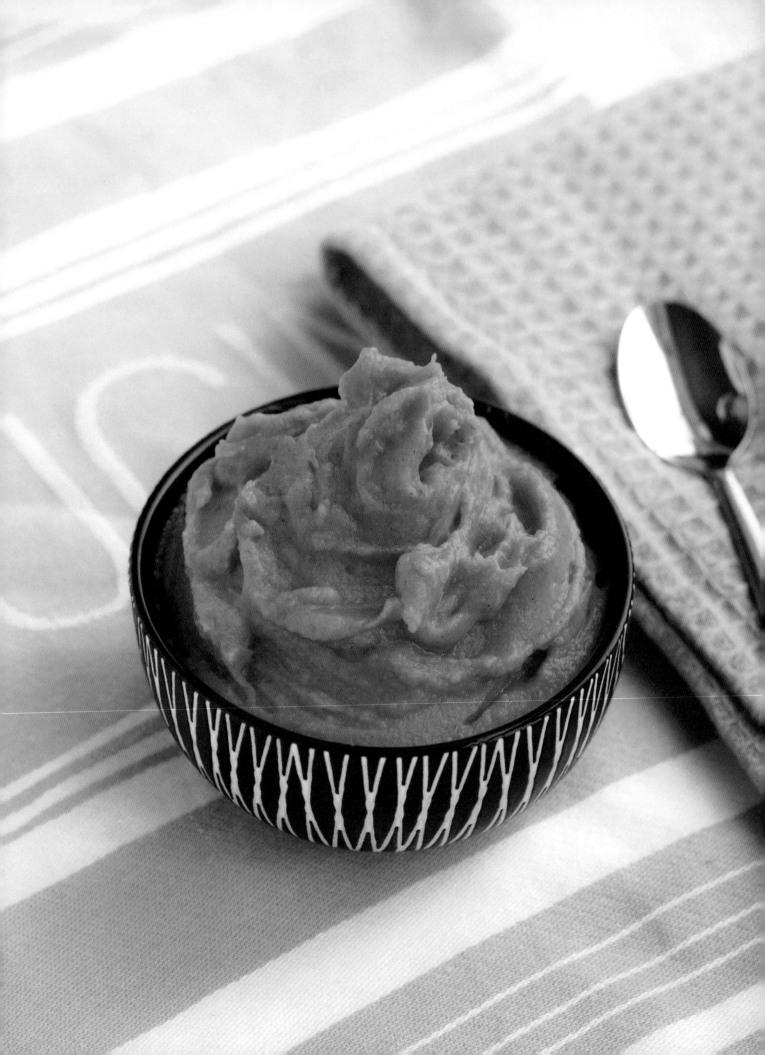

Sweet Potato Pie Ice Cream

PREP TIME: 5 minutes | **COOK TIME:** 40 minutes | **SERVES:** 1

Ingredients

- 2 medium sweet potatoes
- 3 tbsp unsweetened non-dairy milk
- 1 tbsp pure maple syrup
- 1 tsp cinnamon

WATCH A VIDEO DEMO:

http://bit.ly/potatotreat

Method

If you already have frozen sweet potatoes ready to go skip the first two steps.

Preheat oven to 420°F. Place the sweet potatoes on a parchment-lined baking sheet, untouched (do not pierce) and bake for 40 minutes or until soft. Let cool to room temperature.

Remove the skins, cut into cubes and place in the freezer in an airtight container overnight.

Remove frozen sweet potato chunks from the freezer and let sit, at room temperature for 5-10 minutes, they should be frozen but not rock solid. Place non-dairy milk, cinnamon, maple syrup and sweet potato in your Vitamix.

Secure the Vitamix lid and with the tamper inserted. Blend with a low to medium speed while continuously pushing the mixture down with a tamper, until smooth and creamy. Serve immediately.

NO VITAMIX? Alternatively you can use a food processor or other high powered blender by adding a little extra non-dairy milk as needed. You may need to power off, remove lid and press the mixture down with a spatula, and repeat.

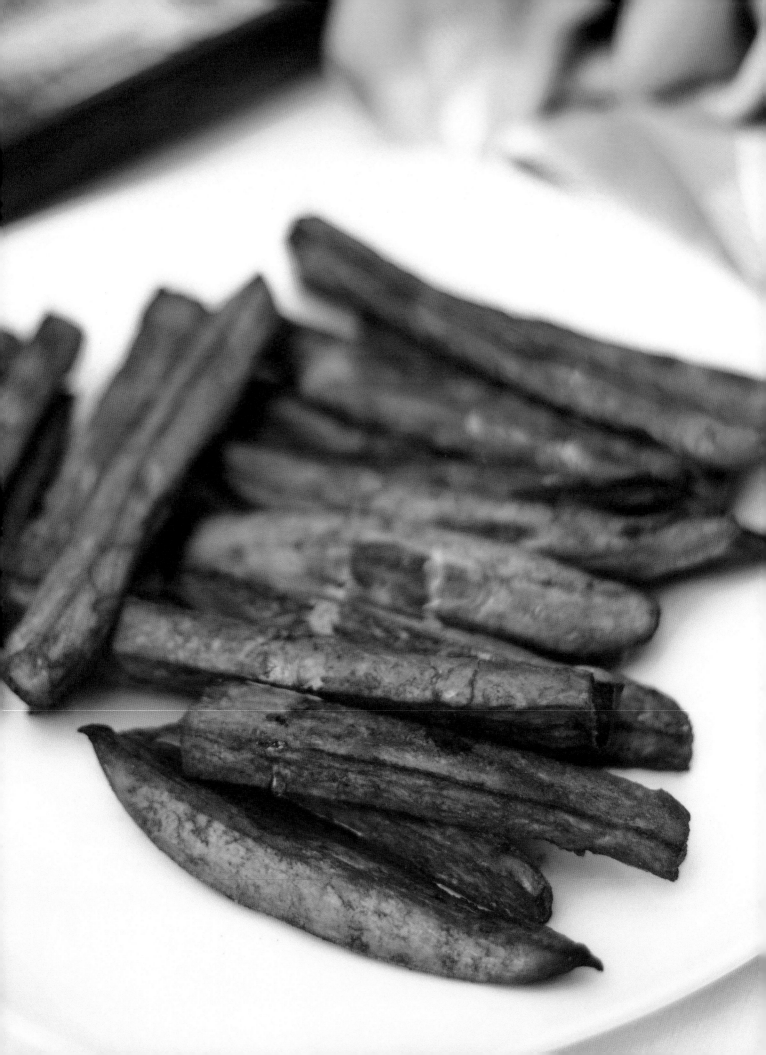

French Toast Sticks

PREP TIME: 5 minutes | **COOK TIME: 40 minutes** | **SERVES: 1**

Ingredients

- 2   sweet potatoes
- 2   tbsp balsamic vinegar
- 1½   tbsp maple syrup
- ½   tbsp maple syrup for topping
- ½   tsp cinnamon

Good With

Herbal tea

Method

Whether you're trying to get through the first 3 days of The Potato Reset, experiencing stress or hormonal cravings, this will provide you with the perfect amount of sweetness to tackle those sugar cravings without over-stimulating your taste buds.

Preheat oven to 400°F. Line a baking sheet with parchment paper. Peel and slice sweet potatoes into thick sticks.

In a large bowl whisk the balsamic vinegar, 1 ½ the tablespoon maple syrup and cinnamon.

Toss sweet potato sticks in the bowl until well coated, then place each stick on the parchment lined baking sheet. Bake for 20 minutes. Flip and bake for another 20 minutes or until desired crispness.

Drizzle with remaining ½ tbsp maple syrup. Serve and enjoy!

Frequently Asked Questions

How many potatoes should I eat?
As many as you need to feel satisfied and not overly full. That number varies person to person, depending on their age and activity level. Test this out! Try a few recipes from this book before you officially start to get an idea of how much you will eat.

How many calories do I need?
This varies person to person, depending on your age, height and activity level. And, it can vary day to day. A sedentary woman in her 50s might only need 1200 calories. An active woman in her 20s might need 2600 calories. This plan is meant to teach you to trust your body to know how much it needs. If you're feeling hungry and not as energetic, chances are you need to eat a little more.

How much weight will I lose per week?
This varies person to person, depending on a lot of factors—age, sex, dieting history, and how much extra weight you have on your body. The more extra weight you have on your body, the quicker you are likely to lose in the beginning. Those coming from an eating-disordered background of restriction may gain in the beginning. If you're currently eating a highly-processed diet, you will find you drop a lot of water weight in the first week. A healthy rate of weight loss is 0.5 lbs to 2 lbs., which is common on this plan.

What can I eat for snacks?
I was surprised that I wasn't hungry in between meals, but some people aren't able to eat large meals that keep them full for 5 hours. If you must snack, it's pretty simple: eat potatoes and veggies. It's always a good idea to snack on non-starchy vegetables such as carrots, celery, broccoli, cucumber – whatever you enjoy. If that doesn't cut it for you, have a small potato.

Can athletes do this?
Yes, just make sure you're eating enough to fuel your training sessions – your hunger will determine this for you. However, competitive athletes may find it difficult to get their energy needs met on potatoes and vegetables only – in this case I suggest planning the Potato Reset for a time when you're not in competition-mode.

Won't I gain weight eating potatoes?
It's what you put on your potatoes that determines whether or not you will gain weight. Butter, cheese, and oil are the culprits to giving the potato a bad name. If you follow the plan as indicated, it's not likely you will gain fat. In some cases, if you are on this plan to overcome an eating disorder that involved severe caloric restriction or purging, you will likely gain some weight in the beginning. And, those who come from a low-carb way of eating may find a slight increase on the scale due to your glycogen stores going back up to a healthy and normal level.

Will I gain weight after?

If you go back to eating junky, processed foods, yes. If you continue transition to a whole foods plant based diet, it's very unlikely. This plan is meant to set you up for long-term success.

How long can I do the Potato Reset?

This is entirely up to you and your doctor. Spudfit ate only potatoes for an entire year and came out healthier than when he started. This did not feel right for me, so I did potatoes only for a month then potatoes and vegetables for a few months before reintroducing other plant foods back into my diet. I recommend one month to get the full benefit, then reassess and decide how much longer you would like to continue.

Can I do this while pregnant or nursing?

I can't recommend this during pregnancy. This could be stressful on your body especially if it's a drastic change to how you normally eat. By cutting out a variety of foods you could miss out on important nutrients. The same goes if you are in the early stages of nursing. Please consult your doctor.

Can I Do this With Diabetes?

Diabetics will need to experiment with their vegetable to potato ratio. Eating sweet potatoes (versus white potatoes) will likely work best, along with more non-starchy vegetables. Depending on how insulin-resistant you are, an abundance of starch at one sitting might not allow for the proper

time needed to process the glucose in your bloodstream. Again, test and see if this is feasible for you.

Can I Do this With Hashimoto's / Lupus / RA and other Autoimmune conditions?

Yes! Many people with autoimmune conditions do well on this plan due to the elimination of inflammatory foods. Any diet high in whole plant foods is helpful for autoimmune conditions. If you are sensitive to white potatoes, you can simply do this plan on sweet potatoes.

Why no dairy?

Whether it comes from a nice small farm or factory farm, being a dairy cow is not a good life. A great video to watch is Dairy Is Scary, a five minute video on YouTube by Erin Janus. To learn about the environmental impact, I highly recommend the documentary "Cowspiracy" on Netflix.

Dairy is also highly addictive due to casomorphins, an opioid compound, that is formed in our stomachs when we consume dairy. Then you add salt into the mix and you might have an idea why it's so difficult to give up cheese. I highly recommend this video by Dr. Barnard: What The Dairy Industry Doesn't Want You to Know.

It's very calorically dense and not as filling as a potato. Then there's a long list of health implications such as osteoporosis, cardiovascular disease and increased risk for various cancers, source: Health Conerns about Dairy Products.

After The Potato Reset

What happens after the Potato Reset?
Instead of going back to your old ways of eating, I recommend transitioning to a whole foods plant-based diet. You've done the work to get the junk out of your system and now your taste buds will appreciate real food. Fruit, and even some vegetables, will taste like candy. You can still continue losing weight when adding a variety of whole plant foods into your diet, such as beans, rice, fruit and a small amount of healthy fats, such as nuts, seeds and avocado.

Start with Fruit
Start the transition process by introducing fruit back into your diet, one serving per day. If you have a history of digestive issues, I recommend introducing one fruit at a time – no closer than three days apart. This will help identify any food sensitivities that you might have.

Other Starches
After a week of adding fruit back in, try replacing one of your potato meals with another starch, such as beans, rice, quinoa or steel cut oats. Again, if you have a history of digestive issues, introduce one new starch every three days.

Whole Plant Fats
Lastly, if you feel you want to reintroduce fats into your diet, keep them to the minimum if you are still wanting to lose weight. Some people do better with some fats in their diet and some may do better without. It's up to you to figure out works best for you and what you are comfortable with. I personally know a few people who can't have nuts around them without risking a binge-eating episode. Some examples of healthy whole plant fats: avocado, walnuts, Brazil nuts, almonds, pumpkin seeds, chia seeds, ground flax seeds, and sesame seeds.

Find a Plan That Works for You
There are many eating styles available as a plant-based eater. Some ways include more fats than others, some more fruit than others, some more starch, and some more raw. Whatever you feel drawn to, go ahead and try it! One of my favorites is High Carb Hannah's Lean & Clean eBook; it's very well balanced with starch as the focus and also includes some healthy fats.

Recommended Resources

Potato Articles

"Potatoes Are Pillars of Worldwide Nutrition"
drmcdougall.com

"The Potato Diet is a Calorie Savings Account"
criticalmas.com

"Potatoes: Man's Best Friend (Not Worst Enemy!)"
ucdintegrativemedicine.com

"The Guy Who Ate Potatoes-Only For One Year"
spudfit.com

YouTube Videos

Potato Wisdom "Potato Diet 12 Week Results"
High Carb Hannah "30 Day Potato Cleanse Results"
Dr. Lisle "The Cram Circuit - The Story of Overeating"
Dr. Lisle "The Pleasure Trap - How to Beat Food Addictions"
Chef AJ "Fat Vegan to Skinny Bitch"
Chef AJ "What Chef AJ Eats in a Day"

Recipe Websites

brandnewvegan.com
mrsplantintexas.com
rawtillwhenever.com
straightupfood.com
thevegan8.com
plantpoweredkitchen.com

Recipe Books

Starch Solution, Dr. McDougall
Lean & Clean, High Carb Hannah
Straight Up Food, Cathy Fisher
Unprocessed, Chef AJ

Educational Books

The Cheese Trap, Neal Barnard
The China Study, T. Collin Campbell
How Not to Die, Dr. Greger
The Pleasure Trap, Dr. Lisle & Dr. Goldhamer
Whole, T. Collin Campbell

Educational Documentaries

Forks Over Knives
Cowspiracy
What the Health
Eating You Alive

About the Author

Jeannine Elder is a graphic designer, illustrator and YouTuber on a mission to empower women and men in their health journey, reach their ideal weight without feeling hangry and lead them to a healthy whole foods plant based way of eating.

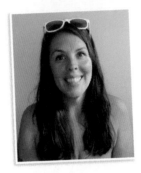

In an effort to simplify and prove once and for all that a carbohydrate-rich diet does not cause weight gain, in February 2017, Jeannine ate only potatoes for an entire month and as a result, lost 8 pounds, diminished junk food cravings and reset her taste buds.

She's been a junk foodie her entire life which ultimately lead to health complications in her early 30s – eczema, gallstones and severe hypothyroidism due to Hashimoto's disease.

Jeannine and her husband Scott switched to a vegan diet on May 21, 2011 after watching the documentary Forks Over Knives. But it wasn't until she focused more on whole foods that she felt a significant increase in energy and overall well being.

Since then she has lost over 40 pounds eating a potato-based diet and inspired many others to do the same. She has helped women with autoimmune conditions realize that they too can reach their healthy weight with the power of the potato.

Jeannine offers one-on-one and group potato coaching for those that need a little extra help or accountability. She currently resides in Cambridge, Ontario, Canada.

Connect with Jeannine

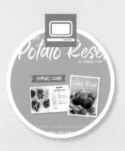

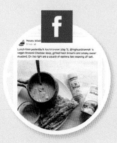

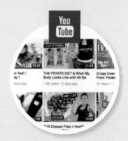

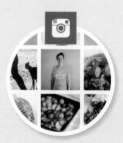

Website: potatoreset.com

facebook.com/ potatowise

youtube.com/c/ potatowisdom

Instagram: @potato.wisdom

Printed in Poland
by Amazon Fulfillment
Poland Sp. z o.o., Wrocław

42232600R00058